T0261763

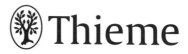

Lung Cancer Screening

Mark S. Parker, MD, FACR
Professor
Diagnostic Radiology and Internal Medicine
Director
Thoracic Imaging Division
Director
Thoracic Imaging Fellowship Program
Director
Lung Cancer Screening Program
VCU Health
Richmond, Virginia

Robert C. Groves, MD
Associate Program Director
Radiology Residency Program
Assistant Professor of Radiology
Cardiothoracic Division
Department of Radiology
VCU Health
Richmond, Virginia

Joanna E. Kusmirek, MD
Assistant Professor of Radiology
Cardiothoracic Division
Department of Radiology
VCU Health
Richmond, Virginia

Leila Rezai Gharai, MD
Assistant Professor of Radiology
Cardiothoracic Division
Department of Radiology
VCU Health
Richmond, Virginia

Samira Shojaee, MD
Assistant Professor of Internal Medicine
Fellowship Director
Interventional Pulmonology
Division of Pulmonary and Critical Care Medicine
VCU Health
Richmond, Virginia

52 illustrations

Thieme
New York • Stuttgart • Delhi • Rio de Janeiro

Executive Editor: William Lamsback
Managing Editor: Haley Paskalides
Director, Editorial Services: Mary Jo Casey
Production Editor: Naamah Schwartz
International Production Director: Andreas Schabert
Editorial Director: Sue Hodgson
International Marketing Director: Fiona Henderson
International Sales Director: Louisa Turrell
Director of Sales, North America: Mike Roseman
Senior Vice President and Chief Operating Officer:
  Sarah Vanderbilt
President: Brian D. Scanlan

Library of Congress Cataloging-in-Publication Data

Names: Parker, Mark S., author.
Title: Lung cancer screening / Mark S. Parker, MD, FACR,
  Professor, Diagnostic Radiology and Internal Medicine,
  Director, Thoracic Imaging Division, Director, Thoracic
  Imaging Fellowship Program, Director, Lung Cancer
  Screening Program, VCU Health, Richmond, VA, United
  States, Robert C. Groves, MD, Associate Program Director,
  Radiology Residency Program, Assistant Professor of
  Radiology, Cardiothoracic Division, Department of Radi-
  ology, VCU Health, Richmond, VA, United States, Joanna E.
  Kusmirek, MD, Assistant Professor of Radiology, Cardio-
  thoracic Division, Department of Radiology, VCU Health,
  Richmond, VA, United States, Leila Rezai Gharai, MD,
  Assistant Professor of Radiology, Cardiothoracic Division,
  Department of Radiology, VCU Health, Richmond, VA,
  United States, Samira Shojaee, MD, Assistant Professor of
  Internal Medicine, Fellowship Director, Interventional
  Pulmonology, Pulmonary and Critical Care Medicine,
  VCU Health, Richmond, VA, United States.
Description: New York : Thieme, [2018] | Includes
  bibliographical references.
Identifiers: LCCN 2017042987| ISBN 9781626235137
  (print) | ISBN 9781626235144 (ebook)
Subjects: LCSH: Lungs–Cancer–Diagnosis. |
  Lungs–Tomography.
Classification: LCC RC280.L8 P36 2018 | DDC 616.99/
  424075–dc23 LC record available at https://lccn.loc.gov/
  2017042987

Thieme Publishers New York
333 Seventh Avenue, New York, NY 10001 USA
+1 800 782 3488, customerservice@thieme.com

Thieme Publishers Stuttgart
Rüdigerstrasse 14, 70469 Stuttgart, Germany
+49 [0]711 8931 421, customerservice@thieme.de

Thieme Publishers Delhi
A-12, Second Floor, Sector-2, Noida-201301
Uttar Pradesh, India
+91 120 45 566 00, customerservice@thieme.in

Thieme Revinter Publicações Ltda.
Rua do Matoso, 170
Rio de Janeiro, RJ, CEP 20270-135, Brasil
+55 21 2563 9700

Cover design: Thieme Publishing Group
Typesetting by Thomson Digital, India

Printed in India by Replika Press Pvt Ltd   5 4 3 2 1

ISBN 978-1-62623-513-7

Also available as an e-book:
eISBN 978-1-62623-514-4

Important note: Medicine is an ever-changing science undergoing continual development. Research and clinical experience are continually expanding our knowledge, in particular our knowledge of proper treatment and drug therapy. Insofar as this book mentions any dosage or application, readers may rest assured that the authors, editors, and publishers have made every effort to ensure that such references are in accordance with **the state of knowledge at the time of production of the book.**

Nevertheless, this does not involve, imply, or express any guarantee or responsibility on the part of the publishers in respect to any dosage instructions and forms of applications stated in the book. **Every user is requested to examine carefully** the manufacturers' leaflets accompanying each drug and to check, if necessary in consultation with a physician or specialist, whether the dosage schedules mentioned therein or the contraindications stated by the manufacturers differ from the statements made in the present book. Such examination is particularly important with drugs that are either rarely used or have been newly released on the market. Every dosage schedule or every form of application used is entirely at the user's own risk and responsibility. The authors and publishers request every user to report to the publishers any discrepancies or inaccuracies noticed. If errors in this work are found after publication, errata will be posted at www.thieme.com on the product description page.

Some of the product names, patents, and registered designs referred to in this book are in fact registered trademarks or proprietary names even though specific reference to this fact is not always made in the text. Therefore, the appearance of a name without designation as proprietary is not to be construed as a representation by the publisher that it is in the public domain.

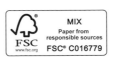

To Cindy, my beautiful, loving, and supportive wife, for always being there by my side.

—Mark S. Parker

To my family for their endless support.

—Leila Rezai Gharai

Lung cancer is NOT a self-inflicted disease. As health care professionals, we all need to strive to abolish this public and sometimes personal misperception and the unfair stigma associated with this often-lethal disease. A person no more deserves to have lung cancer because he or she once smoked or currently smokes than does a person deserve to have a car accident simply because he or she owns and drives a car.

Mark S. Parker, MD, FACR

Contents

Preface

Lung cancer is the leading cause of cancer death for both men and women, not only in the United States but also worldwide. Each and every day of the week, lung cancer alone kills more Americans than all of the cancers of the breast, prostate, colorectum, liver, kidney, and melanoma combined. Among the top four deadliest cancers in the United States (lung, prostate, breast, and colorectal), lung cancer has been the only cancer not subject to routine screening. Historically, this reflected the fact that no screening test (e.g., chest radiography, sputum cytology) had ever been shown to reduce lung cancer–specific mortality. However, this fact dramatically changed with the release of the National Lung Screening Trial (NLST) results in November 2011. This randomized control trial showed that high-risk persons receiving a baseline and subsequent annual low-dose lung cancer screening computed tomographies (CTs) had a 20% lower risk of death from lung cancer compared to individuals screened with conventional radiography. This was the first time in the history of medicine that physicians finally had a screening test available that could dramatically impact the lives of thousands upon thousands of persons at risk for this otherwise lethal disease. Since the release of the NLST results, gradually more and more medical societies and organizations have come on board to recognize the role and impact of lung cancer screening on the early detection of lung cancer. At last count, more than 40 such societies and organizations have endorsed lung cancer screening in high-risk persons. More recently, both the U.S. Preventive Services Task Force (USPSTF) and the Centers for Medicare & Medicaid Services (CMS) have endorsed lung cancer screening in eligible high-risk persons. Due to the rapid evolution of lung cancer screening CT, many primary health care providers and radiologists alike are uncertain of the eligibility criteria for screening. Many are likewise unfamiliar with the benefits and potential harms associated with mass lung cancer screening programs, including the false-positive, false-negative, and overdiagnosis rates associated with lung cancer screening, and the radiation dose exposure associated with such and how to formally report and manage the lung cancer–specific and incidental imaging findings detected on these screening CT examinations. Addressing each of these issues is the goal and purpose of this textbook.

Mark S. Parker, MD, FACR

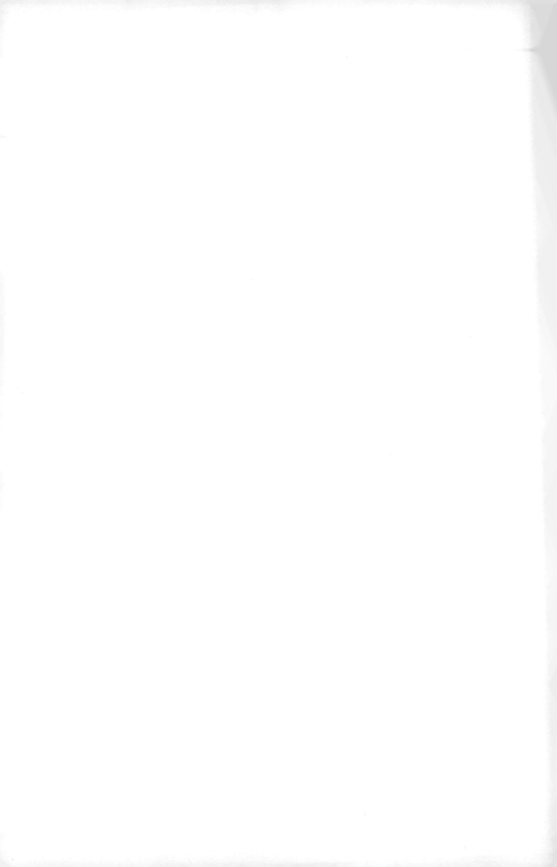

Contributors

Michelle Futrell, MSN, MBA, RN
Clinical Nurse III
Program Coordinator
Lung Cancer Screening
Department of Radiology
VCU Health
Richmond, Virginia

Leila Rezai Gharai, MD
Assistant Professor of Radiology
Cardiothoracic Division
Department of Radiology
VCU Health
Richmond, Virginia

Robert C. Groves, MD
Associate Program Director
Radiology Residency Program
Assistant Professor of Radiology
Cardiothoracic Division
Department of Radiology
VCU Health
Richmond, Virginia

Joanna E. Kusmirek, MD
Assistant Professor of Radiology
Cardiothoracic Division
Department of Radiology
VCU Health
Richmond, Virginia

Peter M.J. Lee, MD
Director of Bronchoscopy & Interventional
    Pulmonology
Hunter-Holmes McGuire VA Medical Center
Richmond, Virginia

Mark S. Parker, MD, FACR
Professor
Diagnostic Radiology and Internal Medicine
Director
Thoracic Imaging Division
Director
Thoracic Imaging Fellowship Program
Director
Lung Cancer Screening Program
VCU Health
Richmond, Virginia

Avinash Pillutla, MD
Diagnostic Radiology Resident (Post-Graduate
    Year 2)
Virginia Commonwealth University Hospital
    System
Glen Allen, Virginia

Deepankar Sharma, MD
Interventional Pulmonology Fellow
Virginia Commonwealth University
North Chesterfield, Virginia

Samira Shojaee, MD
Assistant Professor of Internal Medicine
Fellowship Director
Interventional Pulmonology
Division of Pulmonary and Critical Care Medicine
VCU Health
Richmond, Virginia

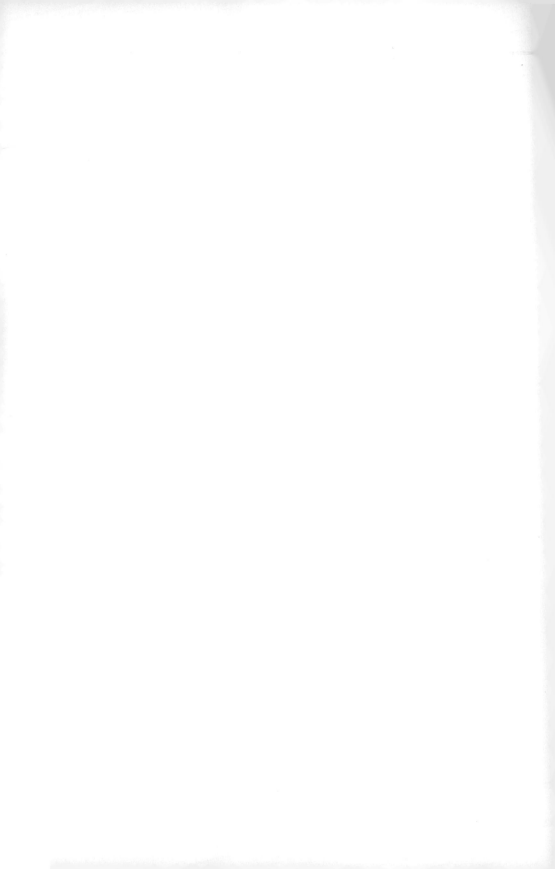

1 Lung Cancer Epidemiology

Mark S. Parker

Summary
This chapter discusses the epidemiology of lung cancer both globally and in the United States including the number of new diagnoses and expected deaths from lung cancer in 2017. A cost analysis of the impact of cancer and lung cancer in particular on society is also addressed.

Keywords: lung cancer, epidemiology, new diagnoses, new deaths, age-adjusted death rates, LIVESTRONG, global impact, economic loss

1.1 Introduction

Lung cancer is the leading cause of cancer death for both men and women, not only in the United States, but also worldwide. Lung cancer alone accounts for about 27% of all cancer deaths in the United States. Each year, in the United States, lung cancer claims the lives of more men and women than all of the cancers of the breast, prostate, colorectum, kidney, and melanoma combined.

Worldwide in 2012, the latest year for which global statistics are available, new cases of lung cancer were diagnosed in more than 1.8 million men and women, comprising 13% of all new cancer diagnoses (▶ Fig. 1.1). More than 1.6 million men and women died of this disease. That is, lung cancer was responsible for 19% of all cancer-related deaths in the world (▶ Fig. 1.2).

In the United States, the American Cancer Society estimates that in 2017, over 222,500 new diagnoses of lung cancer will be made. This includes about 116,990 American men and 105,510 American women. The American Cancer Society further estimates that in 2017, about 155,870 Americans will die from lung cancer, including roughly 84,590 men and 71,280 women.

The age-adjusted death rate for lung cancer is higher for men (51.7 per 100,000 persons) than for women (34.7 per 100,000 persons). It is similar for African Americans (45.7 per 100,000 persons) and Caucasians (45.4 per 100,000 persons). However, African American men have a far higher age-adjusted lung cancer death rate than Caucasian men, while African American and Caucasian women have similar rates.

To put these statistics into perspective, realize that *one new diagnosis* of lung cancer is made *EVERY 2.5 minutes*, and that *one person dies* from lung cancer *EVERY 3 minutes* in the United States alone.

1.2 Cost Analysis and Impact on Society

Cancer is the world's leading cause of death, followed by heart disease and stroke. The American Cancer Society and LIVESTRONG conducted a landmark study assessing the economic cost of all causes of death globally. Their results showed that cancer has the greatest and most devastating economic impact from premature death and disability of any cause of death in the world.

Globally, in 2008, the latest year for which worldwide statistics are available, the total economic impact of premature death, disability, and lost years of life and productivity

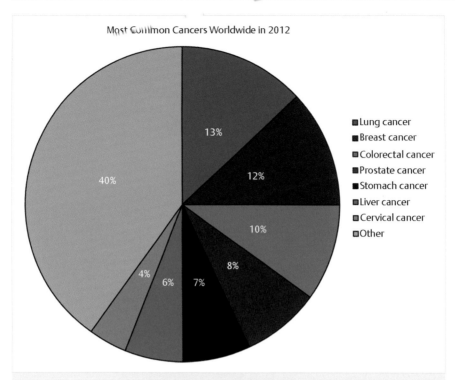

Fig. 1.1 Most common cancers worldwide. (Adapted with permission from "Most Common Cancers Worldwide in 2012" and "Most Common Causes of Cancer Death Worldwide in 2012": http://www.cdc.gov/cancer/international/statistics.htm.)

from cancer worldwide was $895 billion. This dollar amount represents 1.5% of the world's gross domestic product (GDP). Deaths and disability from lung cancer, colorectal cancer, and breast cancer account for the largest economic costs globally. More specifically, the global economic impact of lung cancer is $188 billion dollars, colorectal cancer $99 billion, and breast cancer $88 billion. The economic toll from cancer is nearly 19% higher than heart disease, the second leading cause ($753 billion). It should be emphasized that this particular analysis did not include direct medical costs, which would further increase the total economic cost of cancer compared to other causes of death. Much of this economic loss stems from the fact that cigarette smokers die on average 15 years earlier than nonsmokers. It is estimated that if the current trend continues, tobacco will be responsible for the death of 7 million persons annually by 2020 and 8 million persons by 2030. Eighty percent of these deaths will occur in low- to middle-income countries and one-third of these deaths will be from cancer.

In comparison to other countries around the world, the United States experiences the biggest economic loss in absolute dollars from cancer, approximately 1.73% of its GDP. The National Institutes of Health (NIH) estimates that cancer care cost the United States an overall $147.5 billion in 2015, $13.4 billion of which was due to lung cancer. Lost productivity due to early death from cancer led to an additional cost of $134.8 billion in 2005, $36.1 billion of which was caused by lung cancer. In 2005, lung cancer was responsible for 2.4 million person-years of life lost. By definition, person-years of

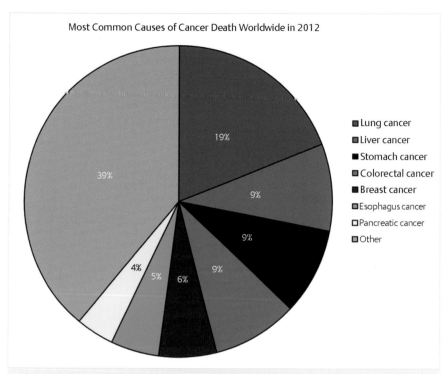

Fig. 1.2 Most common cancer deaths worldwide. (Adapted with permission from "Most Common Cancers Worldwide in 2012" and "Most Common Causes of Cancer Death Worldwide in 2012": http://www.cdc.gov/cancer/international/statistics.htm.)

life lost is the difference between the actual age at death due to the disease and the expected age of death in the absence of the disease. Compared with other cancers, lung cancer far exceeds the number of persons-years-of-life lost. The economic toll associated with these lost years of life is staggering. One study published in 2000 estimated these costs at $289.4 billion. Furthermore, the direct medical costs related to lung cancer treatment in 2004 were estimated at $9.6 billion. Direct medical costs include services patients receive, including but not limited to hospitalization(s), surgery, office visits, radiation therapy, and chemotherapy/immunotherapy. Such costs are typically measured by insurance payments and patient's out-of-pocket co-payments and deductibles. Indirect costs of cancer are more difficult to accurately quantitate and include the monetary losses associated with time spent receiving medical care, lost time from the job, and loss of productivity due to premature death. These latter costs are incurred not only by the affected patient(s), but also by their caregivers and family members.

Suggested Readings

[1] American Cancer Society. Cancer Facts and Figures 2016. Available at: http://www.cancer.org/acs/groups/content/@research/documents/document/acspc-047079.pdf. Accessed June 12, 2016

[2] American Cancer Society. Table 1. Estimated Number of New Cancer Cases and Deaths by Sex, US, 2017: Cancer Facts and Figures 2017. Available at: https://www.cancer.org/content/dam/cancer-org/research/

cancer-facts-and-statistics/annual-cancer-facts-and-figures/2017/estimated-number-of-new-cancer-cases-and-deaths-by-sex-us-2017.pdf

[3] American Cancer Society. Cancer Facts & Figures 2017. Available at: https://www.cancer.org/research/cancer-facts-statistics/all-cancer-facts-figures/cancer-facts-figures-2017.html

[4] Siegel RL, Miller KD, Jemal A. Cancer statistics, 2017. CA Cancer J Clin 2017;67(1):7–30

[5] Statistics GC. International Cancer Control. Available at: http://www.cdc.gov/cancer/international/statistics.htm. Accessed August 5, 2016

[6] The Global Economic Cost of Cancer. Available at: http://www.cancer.org/acs/groups/content/@internationalaffairs/documents/document/acspc-026203.pdf Accessed August 5, 2016

[7] Lung Cancer Fact Sheet/ American Lung Association. Available at: http://www.lung.org/lung-health-and-diseases/lung-disease-lookup/lung-cancer/learn-about-lung-cancer/lung-cancer-fact-sheet.html Accessed October 26, 2016

[8] Cipriano LE, Romanus D, Earle CC, et al. Lung cancer treatment costs, including patient responsibility, by disease stage and treatment modality, 1992 to 2003. Value Health. 2011; 14(1):41–52

[9] Siegel RL, Miller KD, Jemal A. Cancer statistics, 2016. CA Cancer J Clin. 2016; 66(1):7–30

[10] Surveillance, Epidemiology, and End Results (SEER) Program. SEER*Stat Database: Mortality-All COD, Total US (1969–2014) < Early Release with Vintage 2014 Katrina/Rita Population Adjustment > -Linked To County Attributes-Total US, 1969–2014 Counties. Bethesda, MD: National Cancer Institute, Division of Cancer Control and Population Sciences, Surveillance Research Program, Surveillance Systems Branch; 2016; underlying mortality data provided by National Center for Health Statistics 2016

[11] Surveillance, Epidemiology, and End Results (SEER) Program. SEER*Stat Database: Mortality-All COD, Total US (1990–2014) < Early Release with Vintage 2014 Katrina/Rita Population Adjustment > -Linked To County Attributes-Total US, 1969–2014 Counties. Bethesda, MD: National Cancer Institute, Division of Cancer Control and Population Sciences, Surveillance Research Program, Surveillance Systems Branch; 2016; underlying mortality data provided by National Center for Health Statistics 2016

[12] U.S. National Institutes of Health. National Cancer Institute. Cancer Trends Progress Report – Financial Burden of Cancer Care. Bethesda, MD: NIH, DHHS; 2015

[13] Yabroff KR, Lund J, Kepka D, Mariotto A. Economic burden of cancer in the United States: estimates, projections, and future research. Cancer Epidemiol Biomarkers Prev. 2011; 20(10):2006–2014

2 Risk Factors for Lung Cancer

Mark S. Parker

Summary

This chapter discusses the most common cause of lung cancer, namely, cigarette smoking, and the numerous chemicals and carcinogens found in cigarette smoke. Other well-known and less well-known causative factors are also discussed.

Keywords: lung cancer, cigarettes, radon, secondhand smoke exposure, asbestos and other occupational carcinogens, COPD, interstitial lung disease

2.1 Introduction

Cigarette smoking remains the single most important risk factor for the development of lung cancer. The risk of lung cancer increases with both the quantity and duration of smoking. It is estimated that 10% of heavy smokers will develop lung cancer. Smoking contributes to 80% of lung cancer deaths in women and 90% of such deaths in men. Male heavy smokers are **23 times** more likely to develop lung cancer than nonsmoking men. Female heavy smokers are **13 times** more likely to develop lung cancer than non-smoking women. The relative risk varies between **9- and 10-fold** for average-heavy smokers and the relative risk is greatest for the development of squamous cell and small cell lung cancers (▶ Table 2.1). The relative risk associated with cigar and pipe smoking is about five times that of nonsmokers (▶ Table 2.1).

Table 2.1 Risk factors for the development of lung cancer

Predisposing risk factor	Increased relative risk
Cigarette smoking	9–20×
Cigar/pipe smoking	5×
Secondhand smoke exposure	1.34
Nonsmokers living with smokers	1.1–1.2×
Marijuana	8% per joint year (1 joint/day)
Domestic radon exposure	1.14× (increases with duration of exposure and smoking)
Asbestos exposure	3.5×
Other occupational particulates (e.g., silica, arsenic, nickel, chromium)	1.21×
Air pollution	1.21×
Wood smoke	1.21×
Positive family history lung cancer	2×
Personal history COPD	4× (1% risk/year)
α_1-Antitrypsin deficiency	2×
Interstitial fibrosis	8.25×
HIV/AIDS	3.6×
Other infections	±

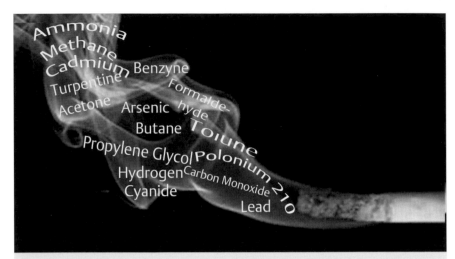

Fig. 2.1 Some of the numerous toxins and poisons present in tobacco smoke emanating from a single cigarette.

Cigarette smoke contains over 7,000 chemicals, about 250 of which are known to be harmful and 70 of which are recognized carcinogens. Cigarette smoke containing carcinogens include polycyclic aromatic hydrocarbons (PAHs), aromatic amines, N-nitrosamines, and other organic and inorganic compounds, such as benzene, vinyl chloride, arsenic, and chromium. Cigarette smoke also contains radioactive compounds, such as radon and its decay products, as well as bismuth and polonium 210. Some of the chemicals and other poisons found in cigarette smoke, which no person would otherwise ever consider ingesting or inhaling, include the following: turpentine (paint thinner), propylene glycol (preservative), butane (lighter fluid), cadmium (used batteries), lead (neurologic toxin), ammonia (household toilet cleaner), benzene (crude oil), formaldehyde (embalming fluid), acetone (finger nail polish remover), arsenic (rat poison), methane (sewer gas), hydrogen cyanide (poison and used in various pesticides), toluene (paint thinners), carbon monoxide (exhaust fumes), etc. Although cigarettes today contain less tar and nicotine, the lower level of nicotine compels smokers to smoke more intensely, drag, puff, or inhale more deeply and frequently. This results in the deposition of carcinogens in the more distal airways and the increased incidence of adenocarcinomas. These chemicals and poisons may be present in each inhaled and exhaled puff of cigarette smoke (▶ Fig. 2.1).

In 2014, nearly 17 of every 100 U.S. adults aged 18 years or older (16.8%) smoked cigarettes. This translates into an estimated 40 million adult smokers. Cigarette smoking is the leading cause of preventable disease and death in the United States, accounting for more than 480,000 deaths every year, or 1 of every 5 deaths.

2.2 Never Smokers

The term *never smokers* refers to those persons who have smoked fewer than 100 cigarettes in their lifetime, including lifetime nonsmokers. Globally, about 15% of lung cancers in men and up to 53% in women are unrelated to cigarette smoking. Never smokers comprise about 25% of all lung cancer cases worldwide. Interestingly, lung cancer in never smokers ranks as the seventh most common cause of cancer death. In South Asia, up to 80% of women with lung cancer are never smokers, whereas in the United States it is estimated that 19% of lung cancer in women and 9% of lung cancer in men occur in never smokers. The age-adjusted rate for lung cancer in never smokers (ages 40–79 years) ranges from 11.2 to 13.7 per 100,000 person-years for men and from 15.2 to 20.8 per 100,000 person-years for women. However, it should be stressed that the rates are 12 to 30 times higher in current smokers of the same age group. The most commonly diagnosed cell type of lung cancer in never smokers is adenocarcinoma.

2.3 Radon

The National Council on Radiation Protection and Measurements recognizes radon and its decay products as being the single largest source of environmental exposure to ionizing radiation among American citizens. Radon is a well-established carcinogen and radon exposure is the *second* most common cause of lung cancer in the United States, responsible for 7,000 to 36,000 lung cancer deaths each year.

Radon-222 is the natural odorless, tasteless, and colorless decay product of radium-226. The latter is the decay product of uranium-238. Both uranium and radium are ubiquitous in the earth's crust found in variable concentrations in the soil, rock, and stone around us. Radon ($t_{1/2} = 3.8$ days) decays into polonium-214 and polonium-218, which emit α-particles that damage the respiratory epithelium when inhaled, causing genetic mutations. The continued decay process eventually forms polonium-210 ($t_{1/2} = 22$ years).

Occupational radon exposure is most frequently encountered in the mining industry. There is a linear relationship between exposure to radon and the risk of developing lung cancer in underground miners. Although uranium mining is no longer taking place in the United States, occupational radon exposure still occurs in the nonuranium mining industry in the United States and in both uranium and nonuranium mines around the world. The Biological Effects of Ionizing Radiation IV study estimated that a 40-year exposure to radon at a concentration above 0.3 work level with an annual cumulative exposure limit of 4 work-level months would increase an exposed individual's lifetime risk of developing lung cancer **twofold**.

Domestic radon exposure is dependent upon the concentration of radon gas in the soil and rock beneath a given dwelling. Other less common sources of domestic radon gas exposure may include the particular home's building materials (e.g., stone, brick, rock), the use of well water and natural gas, and the degree of ventilation in the home. Higher levels of domestic exposure have been reported to have a 1.14 overall relative risk for lung cancer (▶ Table 2.1). However, it has been reported that even a nonsmoker exposed to high levels of radon over a lifetime has a 1 in 20 chance of developing lung cancer. This risk can increase to 1 in 3 for a smoker exposed to high levels of radon over their lifetime. The U.S. Environmental Protection Agency (EPA) estimates the average concentration of radon in American homes to be on the order of 1.25 pCi/L, although there is much variation in levels from home to home. The EPA actionable level is 4 pCi/L. The EPA estimates that 1 in 15 U.S. homes exceeds this actionable level. Home radon gas levels can be easily measured via relatively inexpensive home test kits available through many hardware stores or available online. Certified inspectors can also be contacted to determine the radon level in a given home or living complex.

2.4 Environmental Tobacco Smoke (Secondhand Smoke Exposure)

Environmental tobacco smoke (ETS) is also sometimes referred to as secondhand smoke exposure (SHS). There is a reported dose-dependent relationship between the degree of ETS exposure and the relative risk of developing lung cancer. At least 17% of lung cancers in nonsmokers result from high levels of involuntary ETS exposure during childhood and adolescence. Studies have also revealed a dose-dependent increased risk of lung cancer in nonsmoking women married to men smokers based on the number of cigarettes smoked and the duration of their exposure. In particular, there is up to a 24% excess risk of lung cancer in nonsmokers who live with a cigarette smoker. Another study of nonsmoking women found smoking by their spouse was associated with a 30% excess risk for all cell types of lung cancer. The National Research Council (NRC) reports a 1.34 overall risk of lung cancer associated with ETS or an approximately 30% increased risk for lung cancer in nonsmokers (▶ Table 2.1). The EPA, the U.S. National Toxicology Program, the U.S. Surgeon General, and the International Agency for Research on Cancer have all classified ETS as a known human carcinogen. The American Cancer Society Cancer Prevention Study performed a prospective comparative analysis of 133,835 never smokers living with smoking spouses versus 154,000 never smokers living with nonsmoking spouses. The investigators found the relative risk for lung cancer in women with smoking husbands was 1.2. That is, a 20% increased incidence of lung cancer. Although slightly lower, the relative risk in nonsmoking men living with smoking wives was still elevated at 1.1 (▶ Table 2.1).

There is no risk-free level of ETS. Even brief or limited exposures can be harmful and is associated with an increased incidence of ear infections, sudden infant death syndrome (SIDS), bronchitis, pneumonia, severity and frequency of asthma exacerbations, lung cancer, stroke, and cardiac disease. ETS exposure may also increase the risk of breast cancer, nasal sinus cavity cancer, and nasopharyngeal cancer in adults and leukemia, lymphoma, and some brain tumors in children. Since 1964, approximately 2,500,000 nonsmokers have died from health problems caused by ETS. It is estimated that ETS was responsible for over 300,000 cardiovascular deaths during 2005 to 2009 among adult nonsmokers in the United States alone. Although it is difficult to calculate the precise number of lung cancers resulting from involuntary ETS, it is estimated that approximately 3,000 lung cancer deaths occur each year among adult nonsmokers in the United States as a result of ETS.

Most ETS exposure occurs in either the homes and or workplace. Additional sources of exposure include car vehicles and public places such as bars, restaurants, and casinos. Smoke-free laws are becoming more and more prevalent in public places with the goal of reducing the adverse respiratory and cardiovascular health consequences associated with ETS including cancer among nonsmokers.

2.5 Other Risk Factors

2.5.1 Asbestos

Asbestos exposure is the most widely recognized occupational cause of lung cancer. Asbestos is a naturally occurring fibrous mineral widely utilized in the construction, insulating and braking industries because of its strength, versatility, and fire-retardant qualities. Two distinct types of asbestos fibers have been described: (1) serpentine (chrysotile) and (2) amphibole (amosite, crocidolite, and tremolite). The carcinogenic properties of asbestos have been recognized for decades. The risk of lung cancer in particular is greater for those workers exposed to the amphibole fiber as opposed to the chrysotile fiber. Historically, in the United States, chrysotile has been the most commonly used type of asbestos.

Studies have found that asbestos exposure is associated with an approximate 3.5 increase relative risk for lung cancer after adjusting for age and smoking history (▶ Table 2.1). This increased risk for lung cancer is dose dependent and varies with the fiber type to which the worker is exposed. The risk for lung cancer from nonoccupational asbestos exposure tends to be extremely low. Cigarette smoking potentiates the carcinogenic effect of asbestos. The relative risk for lung cancer with asbestos exposure alone is **sixfold**, with cigarette smoking alone up to **11-fold**, but with exposure to both asbestos and cigarette smoke, the increase has been reported as much as **59-fold**, suggesting a synergistic interaction between the carcinogens of tobacco smoke and asbestos.

2.5.2 Other Potential Occupational Carcinogens

Multiple other agents not infrequently encountered in various industries or occupations have purported carcinogenic effects on the lung (▶ Table 2.1). Some of the potential carcinogens identified by the International Agency for Research on Cancer (IARC) include but are not limited to the following: arsenic (copper, lead, or zinc ore smelting), beryllium (ceramic, electronic and aerospace equipment manufacturing), cadmium (electroplating and plastics industry), chloromethyl ethers (chemical manufacturing), chromium (electroplating and leather tanning), nickel (electroplating, production of stainless and heat-resistant steel, polycyclic aromatics, aluminum production, hydrocarbon compounds, nickel-containing ore smelting, roofing products), radon (mining industry), silica (ceramics, glass foundry, granite, and mining industries), and vinyl chloride (plastics industry). In 2000, it was estimated that 10% of lung cancer deaths among men and 5% of lung cancer deaths among women globally were likely related to exposures to eight occupational lung carcinogens including asbestos, arsenic, beryllium, cadmium, chromium, nickel, silica, and diesel fumes (▶ Table 2.1).

2.5.3 Air Pollution

Air pollution in developing countries continues to impact their society. Not unexpectedly, the highest concentrations of suspected particulate pollutants, sulfur dioxide, and smoke are present in the urban cities of these countries as opposed to more rural settings. Various potential carcinogens are also likely emitted from different sources of fossil fuel combustion, including diesel exhaust. Some of the gaseous components of diesel exhaust include known human carcinogens such as benzene, formaldehyde, and 1,3-butadiene. Such outdoor air pollution has been postulated to heighten the risk for lung cancers. As a corollary, two large independent meta-analyses have demonstrated that occupational exposure to diesel exhaust (e.g., trucking industry) is associated with an approximately 30 to 50% increase relative risk of lung cancer. The data linking a potential association between gasoline engine exhaust fumes and lung cancer are less convincing. Some investigators have described a gradient of relative risk associated with exposure to combustible products. This reported relative risk gradient ranges from 7.0 to 22.0 in cigarette smokers to 1.0 to 1.6 in urban dwellers and 1.0 to 1.5 in nonsmokers exposed to ETS (▶ Table 2.1).

2.5.4 Coal, Crop Residues, and Wood Smoke

Approximately 3 billion people in the world solely depend on solid fuels as their primary source of energy for cooking and heating their homes. Studies have shown an overall 1.29 increase risk for lung cancer in such circumstances (▶ Table 2.1). The IARC recently classified indoor fumes from household coal combustion as a human carcinogen and that from biomass fuels, primarily wood, as a probable human carcinogen. Interestingly, some authorities have reported lung cancer associated with exposure to wood smoke exhibit behavioral patterns similar to those associated with exposure to cigarette smoke.

2.5.5 Chronic Obstructive Lung Disease

Cigarette smoking is the most common cause of both lung cancer and chronic obstructive lung disease (COPD). COPD is characterized by both chronic airway inflammation and chronic airflow obstruction. Both of these latter factors are associated with a statistically significant increased risk of lung cancer in both smokers (**4×**) as well as never smokers (▶ Table 2.1). In fact, COPD is often considered an independent risk factor for lung cancer with a reported 1% risk per year (▶ Table 2.1). COPD affects about 40 to 70% of persons diagnosed with lung cancer. Young et al showed that 50% of 602 patients with lung cancer in their study had prebronchodilator pulmonary function test (PFT) results supporting a concomitant diagnosis of COPD with an OR (odds ratio) of 11.6, independent of age, sex, and smoking history. They found the prevalence of COPD in newly diagnosed lung cancer was **sixfold** greater than in matched smokers. Interestingly, the risk of developing lung cancer may be lower in those with COPD using high-dose inhaled corticosteroids compared with COPD patients who do not routinely use inhaled corticosteroids or only use low-dose steroids. This finding prompted Parimon et al to postulate inhaled corticosteroids may actually have a chemopreventive role against the development of lung cancer in persons with COPD. Yang et al demonstrated that α_1-antitrypsin deficiency carriers also have an increased risk of lung cancer. Adjusting for the effects of cigarette smoking and COPD, they found a **twofold** increased risk of lung cancer in this patient population (▶ Table 2.1).

2.5.6 Interstitial Lung Disease

It is widely recognized that pulmonary fibrosis of many etiologies, including idiopathic pulmonary fibrosis and interstitial lung disease associated with connective tissue disease, is associated with an increased risk of lung cancer. Hubbard et al reported an OR for lung cancer of 8.25 for patients with pulmonary fibrosis after adjusting for smoking compared with controls (▶ Table 2.1). The mechanism by which long-standing fibrosis predisposes to lung cancer has not been identified although the chronic inflammation, recurrent infections, and impaired clearance of potential carcinogens likely play a role.

2.5.7 Family History of Lung Cancer

Various inheritable genetic factors (e.g., high-penetrance, low-frequency genes) undoubtedly play a role in the susceptibility, development, and treatment response of lung cancers in some individuals. This likely is related to their ability to absorb and metabolize various carcinogens present in tobacco smoke and their ability to repair the resultant DNA (deoxyribonucleic acid) damage. The risk is significantly increased for persons with a positive family history of early-onset lung cancer (< 60 years of age). A meta-analysis of 32 studies showed a **twofold** increased risk for lung cancer in persons with such a positive family history (▶ Table 2.1). This increased risk was also observed in nonsmoker family members. As more and more genetic factors and mutations are observed and discovered, this will play more and more of a role in identifying at-risk persons who may benefit from early screening and in the diagnosis and management of lung cancers in the future.

2.5.8 Human Immunodeficiency Virus/Acquired Immune Deficiency Syndrome

The routine use of highly active antiretroviral therapy (HAART) for persons with human immunodeficiency virus/acquired immune deficiency syndrome (HIV/AIDS) has dramatically reduced mortality from this immunodeficiency syndrome. Paradoxically, the combination of HAART and other therapies and the prolongation of life of these individuals have now been accompanied by a proportional increase in the number of deaths from non–AIDS-defining cancers, and from lung cancer in particular. The higher percentage of tobacco abuse in the HIV/AIDS population compared to the non–HIV/AIDS population is likely a contributing factor. Kirk et al showed that after controlling for smoking, HIV infection is associated with a hazard ratio of **3.6** for lung cancer (▶ Table 2.1). However, factors other than cigarette smoking alone likely have contributory roles including the greater prevalence of co-infection with oncogenic viruses (e.g., human herpesvirus-8, human papilloma virus, Epstein–Barr virus) as well as the direct effects of the HIV itself and long-standing immunosuppression. Supporting this hypothesis, it has been well documented that HIV/AIDS–infected cancer patients have a worse prognosis than similarly staged non–HIV/AIDS infected persons with the same cancer type. Additionally, most HIV/AIDS cancer patients will have more advanced disease and reduced median survival at the time of their diagnosis compared to similar noninfected cancer patients. Most of the former individuals will also be younger than the average lung cancer patient at diagnosis, which may contribute to delays in the appropriate diagnosis and management of lung cancer.

Suggested Readings

[1] Aldington S, Harwood M, Cox B, et al. Cannabis and Respiratory Disease Research Group. Cannabis use and risk of lung cancer: a case-control study. Eur Respir J. 2008; 31(2):280–286

[2] Bhatia R, Lopipero P, Smith AH. Diesel exhaust exposure and lung cancer. Epidemiology. 1998; 9(1):84–91

[3] Boffetta P, Pershagen G, Jöckel KH, et al. Cigar and pipe smoking and lung cancer risk: a multicenter study from Europe. J Natl Cancer Inst. 1999; 91(8):697–701

[4] Brenner DR, Hung RJ, Tsao MS, et al. Lung cancer risk in never-smokers: a population-based case-control study of epidemiologic risk factors. BMC Cancer. 2010; 10:285

[5] Bryant A, Cerfolio RJ. Differences in epidemiology, histology, and survival between cigarette smokers and never-smokers who develop non-small cell lung cancer. Chest. 2007; 132(1):185–192

[6] International Agency for Research on Cancer. Involuntary Smoking. Vol. 83. Lyon, France: International Agency for Research on Cancer Monographs; 2002

[7] Cardenas VM, Thun MJ, Austin H, et al. Environmental tobacco smoke and lung cancer mortality in the American Cancer Society's Cancer Prevention Study. II. Cancer Causes Control. 1997; 8(1):57–64

[8] Dela Cruz CS, Tanoue LT, Matthay RA. Lung cancer: epidemiology, etiology, and prevention. Clin Chest Med. 2011; 32(4):605–644

[9] Department of Health and Human Services. The Health Benefits of Smoking Cessation: A Report of the Surgeon General. DHHS Pub. No. (CDC) 90–8416. Washington, DC: US DHHS; 1990

[10] Engels EA, Brock MV, Chen J, Hooker CM, Gillison M, Moore RD. Elevated incidence of lung cancer among HIV-infected individuals. J Clin Oncol. 2006; 24(9):1383–1388

[11] Fabrikant JI. Radon and lung cancer: the BEIR IV Report. Health Phys. 1990; 59(1):89–97

[12] Fontham ET, Correa P, Reynolds P, et al. Environmental tobacco smoke and lung cancer in nonsmoking women. A multicenter study. JAMA. 1994; 271(22):1752–1759

[13] Hackshaw AK, Law MR, Wald NJ. The accumulated evidence on lung cancer and environmental tobacco smoke. BMJ. 1997; 315(7114):980–988

[14] Henley SJ, Thun MJ, Chao A, Calle EE. Association between exclusive pipe smoking and mortality from cancer and other diseases. J Natl Cancer Inst. 2004; 96(11):853–861

[15] Hessel PA, Gamble JF, McDonald JC. Asbestos, asbestosis, and lung cancer: a critical assessment of the epidemiological evidence. Thorax. 2005; 60(5):433–436

[16] Hosgood HD, III, Boffetta P, Greenland S, et al. In-home coal and wood use and lung cancer risk: a pooled analysis of the International Lung Cancer Consortium. Environ Health Perspect. 2010; 118(12):1743–1747

[17] Hubbard R, Venn A, Lewis S, Britton J. Lung cancer and cryptogenic fibrosing alveolitis. A population-based cohort study. Am J Respir Crit Care Med. 2000; 161(1):5–8

[18] Janerich DT, Thompson WD, Varela LR, et al. Lung cancer and exposure to tobacco smoke in the household. N Engl J Med. 1990; 323(10):632–636

[19] Kirk GD, Merlo C, O' Driscoll P, et al. HIV infection is associated with an increased risk for lung cancer, independent of smoking. Clin Infect Dis. 2007; 45(1):103–110

[20] Lavolé A, Wislez M, Antoine M, Mayaud C, Milleron B, Cadranel J. Lung cancer, a new challenge in the HIV-infected population. Lung Cancer. 2006; 51(1):1–11

[21] Le Jeune I, Gribbin J, West J, Smith C, Cullinan P, Hubbard R. The incidence of cancer in patients with idiopathic pulmonary fibrosis and sarcoidosis in the UK. Respir Med. 2007; 101(12):2534–2540

[22] Littman AJ, Jackson LA, Vaughan TL. Chlamydia pneumoniae and lung cancer: epidemiologic evidence. Cancer Epidemiol Biomarkers Prev. 2005; 14(4):773–778

[23] Loganathan RS, Stover DE, Shi W, Venkatraman E. Prevalence of COPD in women compared to men around the time of diagnosis of primary lung cancer. Chest. 2006; 129(5):1305–1312

[24] Lubin JH, Boice JD, Jr. Lung cancer risk from residential radon: meta-analysis of eight epidemiologic studies. J Natl Cancer Inst. 1997; 89(1):49–57

[25] Lubin JH, Boice JD, Jr, Edling C, et al. Lung cancer in radon-exposed miners and estimation of risk from indoor exposure. J Natl Cancer Inst. 1995; 87(11):817–827

[26] Matakidou A, Eisen T, Houlston RS. Systematic review of the relationship between family history and lung cancer risk. Br J Cancer. 2005; 93(7):825–833

[27] National Research Council. Environmental Tobacco Smoke: Measuring Exposures and Assessing Health Effects. Washington, DC: National Academy Press; 1986:337

[28] Nyberg F, Pershagen G. Passive smoking and lung cancer. Accumulated evidence on lung cancer and environmental tobacco smoke. BMJ. 1998; 317(7154):347–348, author reply 348

[29] Parimon T, Chien JW, Bryson CL, McDonell MB, Udris EM, Au DH. Inhaled corticosteroids and risk of lung cancer among patients with chronic obstructive pulmonary disease. Am J Respir Crit Care Med. 2007; 175 (7):712–719

[30] Pope CA, III, Burnett RT, Thun MJ, et al. Lung cancer, cardiopulmonary mortality, and long-term exposure to fine particulate air pollution. JAMA. 2002; 287(9):1132–1141

[31] Saccomanno G, Huth GC, Auerbach O, Kuschner M. Relationship of radioactive radon daughters and cigarette smoking in the genesis of lung cancer in uranium miners. Cancer. 1988; 62(7):1402–1408

[32] Samet JM. Indoor radon and lung cancer: risky or not? J Natl Cancer Inst. 1994; 86(24):1813–1814

[33] Samet JM, Stolwijk J, Rose SL. Summary: international workshop on residential Rn epidemiology. Health Phys. 1991; 60(2):223–227

[34] Spitz MR, Etzel CJ, Dong Q, et al. An expanded risk prediction model for lung cancer. Cancer Prev Res (Phila). 2008; 1(4):250–254

[35] Thorne S, Malarcher A, Maurice M, et al. Centers for Disease Control and Prevention (CDC). Cigarette smoking among adults: United States, 2007. MMWR Morb Mortal Wkly Rep. 2008; 57(45):1221–1226

[36] Thun MJ, Hannan LM, Adams-Campbell LL, et al. Lung cancer occurrence in never-smokers: an analysis of 13 cohorts and 22 cancer registry studies. PLoS Med. 2008; 5(9):e185

[37] US Department of Health and Services. Report of the Surgeon General: The Health Consequences of Involuntary Smoking. (CDC) 87–8398. Washington, DC: DHHS; 1986

[38] US Environmental Protection Agency, Office of Air and Radiation and Office of Research and Development. Respiratory Health Effects of Passive Smoking: Lung Cancer and Other Disorders. EPA/600/6–90/006F. Washington, DC: EPA; 1992

[39] Wakelee HA, Chang ET, Gomez SL, et al. Lung cancer incidence in never smokers. J Clin Oncol. 2007; 25(5): 472–478

[40] Yang P, Sun Z, Krowka MJ, et al. Alpha1-antitrypsin deficiency carriers, tobacco smoke, chronic obstructive pulmonary disease, and lung cancer risk. Arch Intern Med. 2008; 168(10):1097–1103

[41] Yang P. Lung cancer in never smokers. Semin Respir Crit Care Med. 2011; 32(1):10–21

[42] Young RP, Hopkins RJ, Christmas T, Black PN, Metcalf P, Gamble GD. COPD prevalence is increased in lung cancer, independent of age, sex and smoking history. Eur Respir J. 2009; 34(2):380–386

3 Evolution of Lung Cancer Screening

Peter M.J. Lee, Samira Shojaee, and Mark S. Parker

Summary
This chapter discusses the evolution of initial unsuccessful early-detection lung cancer–screening programs with sputum cytology and chest radiography and the reasons for their failure to the current state-of-the-art early detection with LDCT (low-dose computed tomography). The natural history of lung cancer, the National Lung Screening Trials (NLST) results, and the endorsement of lung cancer screening for eligible high-risk persons by the U.S. Preventive Services Task Forces (USPSTF) and the Centers for Medicare & Medicaid Services (CMS) are also addressed.

Keywords: lung cancer, screening, cancer growth, chest radiography, sputum cytology, PLCO, NLST, USPSTF, CMS

3.1 What Is Screening?

Screening means testing for diseases, such as lung cancer, while the individual is still healthy, that is, when there are no symptoms or clinical signs of disease. The purpose of the screen is to find disease early on, when treatment options may be more successful, and individuals may have a much better chance of cure. The intent of lung cancer screening is to detect the disease at its earliest possible stage, while it is small, confined to the thorax and before it invades adjacent tissues, extends beyond the lung, and/or causes symptoms, at which point the chance for cure dramatically diminishes and treatment is less successful. The early detection of lung cancer when it is still small and localized is of paramount importance in mortality reduction. Individuals not infrequently undergo other forms of screening for similar purposes (e.g., blood pressure or cholesterol checks; annual mammography; PAP smear; colonoscopy; PSA; etc.).

3.2 Natural History of Lung Cancer

Unfortunately, lung cancer is a "sneaky" disease. It may harbor in the body for years, growing in size and volume, before becoming large enough to be detectable on a conventional radiograph or before it causes symptoms such as cough, hemoptysis, or weight loss (▶ Fig. 3.1). In the absence of screening, most patients already have locally advanced or metastatic disease when they first see their primary care doctor with these or similar symptoms. Only 15 to 25% of patients have potentially resectable, early-stage disease confined to the chest at that time. Over the years, screening for the early detection of lung cancer has included miniature chest photofluorography, conventional chest radiography, sputum cytology, and more recently low-dose helical computed tomography (CT).

3.3 Chest Radiography

The possibility of tobacco as a primary cause for the increasing incidence of lung cancer was introduced in the early 1900s. The first case control study to highlight this association was from a German scholar, Franz Hermann Müller, in 1939. By the 1950s, several

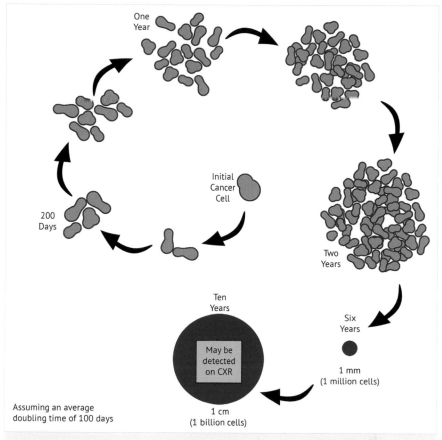

One Year

200 Days

Initial Cancer Cell

Two Years

Ten Years

Six Years

May be detected on CXR

1 mm (1 million cells)

Assuming an average doubling time of 100 days

1 cm (1 billion cells)

Fig. 3.1 Natural history of lung cancer cell growth (Adapted with permission from J. Surg Oncol 1997;65(4):284–297.)

epidemiologic studies further supported this link, concluding smoking 35 cigarettes or more per day increased the odds of death by lung cancer by a factor of 40. Concurrently, in the 1940s, mass screening for tuberculosis began using miniature chest photofluorography or abreugraphy. These early X-ray images were a miniature 50- to 100-mm photograph of the screen of an X-ray fluoroscopy of the thorax and were typically viewed on a projector. Screening with chest radiography was instrumental in the early detection of tuberculosis, leading to early appropriate antimicrobial treatment and improved prognosis. As most thoracic tumors were visible on photofluorography, there was a potential for reducing mortality through screening and early treatment with this modality. Early efforts at screening in the 1950s with several large uncontrolled studies showed mixed results. The earliest U.S.-led studies conducted in the 1950s were the Philadelphia Pulmonary Neoplasm Research Project (PNRP) and a cooperative pilot study between the American Cancer Society and the Veterans Administration (VA). Combined, these two studies enrolled 20,743 males older than 45 years to undergo screening with chest radiography every 6 months with a questionnaire regarding smoking habits, occupation, and respiratory symptoms. A total of 194 screen-detected lung cancers were discovered, but only 35% were resectable. Five-year survival in the PNRP and 32-month survival in the VA cooperative were a disappointing 8% and 17%, respectively. The PNRP was also notable for high (24%) 30-day postoperative mortality rates.

Conversely, two large uncontrolled screening studies in Japan and the United Kingdom suggested some survival benefit. The Tokyo Metropolitan Government study (1,871,374 men and women, all ages) and the South London Lung Cancer Study (67,400 men older than 45 years) showed higher rates of resectability (56%) with improved long-term survival against retrospective comparison groups (44 vs. 20% at 5 years and 18 vs. 9% at 4 years, respectively). Nearly a decade later, two nonrandomized controlled studies conducted in the United Kingdom and Germany were the first to report disease-specific mortality rates. The North London Lung Cancer Study and the Erfurt County Germany Study compared semiannual chest X-ray screening against a control group who received less frequent imaging. While 5-year survival in both studies was superior to the control groups (15 vs. 6% in the UK and 28 vs. 19% in Germany, respectively), there were no differences in mortality rates (0.6–0.8/1,000 persons screened).

By the 1970s, advancements in X-ray technology and imaging processing, sputum cytology techniques, and the flexible fiberoptic bronchoscope generated renewed interest in lung cancer screening using these new modalities. The National Cancer Institute (NCI)—the Mayo Lung Project (MLP), the Johns Hopkins Lung Project (JHLP), and the Memorial Sloan Kettering Lung Project (MSKLP), sponsored three large randomized-control trials (RCT). A fourth RCT was conducted in Czechoslovakia. The MLP and Czechoslovakian studies attempted to assess the efficacy of chest radiography. The JHLP and MSKLP were designed to assess the utility of adding sputum cytology to annual chest X-ray screening. The MLP consisted of men older than 45 years with a history of heavy smoking. After an initial prevalence screen, 9,211 men were subsequently randomized to chest X-ray and sputum screening every 4 months with regular reminders or a control group where annual screening was recommended but without routine reminders. At the end of the study, frequent screening detected a 29% higher incidence of lung cancers compared to the controls (206 vs. 160, respectively). The screened group had a favorable shift toward early-stage tumors (38 vs. 25%, respectively) and higher resectability rates (46 vs. 32%, respectively). Despite an apparent survival advantage in the screened group (33 vs. 15%, respectively), there was no difference in mortality (3.2/1,000 vs. 3.0/1,000 person-years, $p = 0.72$). Notably, there may have been a substantial degree of statistical contamination within the control group—nearly half had obtained annual chest X-rays, with 73% receiving X-rays in the final 2 years.

The Czechoslovakian study screened 6,346 men between the ages of 40 and 64 years. They were randomized to chest X-ray and sputum cytology screening every 6 months for 3 years and a control group who had no testing for 3 years following the prevalence screen. There were 36 screen-detected lung cancers in the study group compared to 19 in the control group with resectability rates of 25 and 16%, respectively. Similar to the MLP, there was an apparent stage shift with favorable 5-year survival in the screened group compared to controls (24 vs. 0%, $p < 0.01$) and no difference in mortality (1.7 vs. 1.5/1,000 person-years).

Despite the proportion of earlier screen-detected lung cancers and apparent survival advantage, these early RCTs were flawed and ultimately incapable of determining whether screening for lung cancer is better than no screening at all. They did not have a proper control group, excluded women, lacked power, and did not consistently report

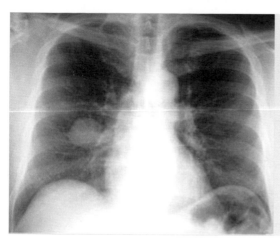

Fig. 3.2 A 40-year-old male patient with hemoptysis. Posteroanterior chest radiograph reveals a 3.0 cm right perihilar mass with well-defined borders. (Reproduced with permission from Hamartoma. In: Parker MS, Rosado-de-Christenson ML, Abbott GF, eds. Chest Imaging Case Atlas. 2nd ed. New York, NY: Thieme; 2012:406-409.)

operative morbidity and mortality. The lack of mortality benefit in the MLP and Czechoslovakian studies was likely influenced by the above factors in addition to biases such as lead time and overdiagnosis. Furthermore, a Cochrane meta-analysis found a relative mortality increase of 11% attributed to frequent lung cancer screening and determined, based on available data, that there was insufficient evidence to recommend lung cancer screening with chest radiography or sputum cytology.

The most recent RCT concerning chest X-ray screening called the Prostate, Lung, Colorectal, and Ovarian (PLCO) trial was conducted to address the statistical flaws in the NCI-sponsored RCTs. Across 10 clinical sites, 154,901 men and women between the ages of 55 and 74 years were randomized to annual screening with posteroanterior (PA) chest X-rays versus usual care for 4 years. Over half were either active or former smokers. Patients were followed for a maximum duration of 13 years. Compliance with screening throughout the study was fair (79–87%) with little contamination in the control arm (11% had imaging). There was no significant difference in lung cancer incidence between groups; however, there were more stage I cancers in the screened versus usual care group (462 vs. 374, respectively). Comparable to the MLP and Czechoslovakian studies, disease-specific lung cancer mortality was similar between groups (relative risk [RR], 0.99; 95% confidence interval [CI], 0.87–1.22; $p = 0.48$).

Thus, screening for the early detection of lung cancer with conventional radiography has not been widely accepted. Screening with conventional radiography is low-yield and has not been proven to reduce patient-specific mortality. In part, this is likely related to difficulty in perceiving upper lobe lesions often silhouetted by overlapping osseous structures such as the anterior and posterior ribs and clavicles, differentiating central hilar lesions from the normal hilar anatomy, and difficulty in perceiving nodules below a threshold of 1 to 2 cm, at which point more than 1 billion cells are already present (▶ Fig. 3.1; ▶ Fig. 3.2).

3.4 Sputum Cytology

Prior to the 1960s, sputum cytology was performed on fresh sputum samples using a "pick-and-smear" technique. This labor-intensive sputum analysis technique was fraught with sampling errors and proved unreliable. In the late 1960s, Saccomanno

17

et al developed a method to both preserve and concentrate sputum samples in a solution of 50% ethyl alcohol and 2% Carbowax®. This solution provided a stable preservation medium for both individual and/or pooled sputum samples and proved valuable in tracking respiratory epithelial atypia and eventual transformation to carcinoma among uranium miners in the western United States. The utility of sputum cytology in the early detection of lung cancer and as a potential screening test was later studied in the 1970s in an NCI-sponsored RCT. The MSKLP and JHLP also investigated the value of adding sputum cytology to regular chest X-ray screening. In these latter investigations, men older than 45 years were randomized into two arms: dual screening with annual chest X-ray and quarterly sputum cytology versus annual chest X-ray screening alone. In toto, 10,194 men received dual screens and 10,232 men received only annual chest X-rays. The investigators found the same incidence of lung cancer in both arms of the investigation. Not surprisingly, most of the lung cancers detected by sputum cytology were of the squamous cell variety (52 of 60). In all, 222 lung cancers were detected in the chest X-ray–only arm, with all major lung cancer cellular subtypes represented. A 9-year follow-up analysis showed lung cancer mortality was slightly lower in the dual-screen population compared with the chest X-ray–only group (RR 0.88; 95% CI, 0.74–1.05). Reductions in mortality were seen for squamous cell cancer deaths (RR, 0.79; 95% CI, 0.54–1.14) and in the heaviest smokers (RR, 0.81; 95% CI, 0.67–1.00). The investigators concluded the data suggested a modest benefit of sputum cytology screening. Respective 5-year and 8-year survival in the MSKLP and JHLP, however, were similar to their control groups (35% in MSKLP and 20% in JHLP). Furthermore, there were no differences in mortality rates (MSKLP: 2.7 vs. 2.7/1,000 person-years; JHLP: 3.4 vs. 3.8/1,000 person-years). The results of these two RCTs have shown no additional benefit to sputum cytology. Two other RCTs, MLP and the Czechoslovakian studies, did not show an overwhelming amount of primary lung cancers detected by sputum analysis (17 and 2, respectively). However, these trials were not designed to assess the efficacy of sputum cytology as a screening method. Due to the lack of positive studies, current guidelines do not recommend using sputum cytology for screening purposes or for the early detection of lung cancer.

3.5 National Lung Screening Trial Results

Lung cancer is the leading cause of cancer death in the United States and worldwide. Despite this fact, among the top four deadliest cancers in the world (i.e., lung, breast, colorectal, and prostate), until just recently, lung cancer was the only major cancer killer not subject to routine screening. Historically, this stemmed from scientific evidence that no early detection program had shown a reduction in patient mortality from lung cancer with sputum and/or conventional radiographic screening. Both practicing physicians and patients at risk for this otherwise lethal disease desperately needed a screening exam for the early detection of lung cancer. After all, this is not an unprecedented concept. The merits of early detection screening programs for other malignancies such as breast and colon cancer are well established clinically. For example, early detection of breast cancer using mammography has resulted in a 5-year survival rate of 90%. Likewise, screening for colorectal cancer has contributed to increased 5-year survival rates of almost 64%.

The prospects for a clinically available definitive early detection lung cancer–screening test changed dramatically when the NCI announced the initial results of the NLST results. The NLST is the largest randomized control trial of lung cancer screening in high-risk persons to date. It was conducted at 33 medical centers across the United States and included more than 53,000 high-risk asymptomatic current or former smokers between the ages of 55 and 74 years with at least a 30-pack-year history of smoking. The $240 million trial, sponsored by the NCI and conducted by the American College of Radiology Imaging Network (ACRIN), showed that high-risk persons who received a baseline and subsequent annual chest low-dose computed tomography (LDCT) scans had a 20% lower risk of death from lung cancer than participants who received standard chest X-ray screening. LDCT detected more lung cancers at earlier and potentially more treatable stages, and it also reduced the number of lung cancer deaths in high-risk persons. This was groundbreaking news because this was the first time in the history of medicine that there was finally a screen available that could positively impact the lives of thousands upon thousands of persons at risk of this disease.

3.6 United States Preventive Services Task Force

Since the release of the NLST results, nearly 40 major medical societies and organizations have endorsed LDCT for the early detection of lung cancer. Notable societies and organizations include the American Lung Association (ALA), American College of Chest Physicians (ACCP), American Society of Clinical Oncology (ASCO), National Comprehensive Cancer Network (NCCN), American Cancer Society (ACS), Lung Cancer Alliance (LCA), and the American Association for Thoracic Surgery (AATS). This culminated in the eventual endorsement of LDCT for the early detection of lung cancer by the U.S. Preventive Services Task Force (USPSTF). The USPSTF is an independent panel of non-federal experts in preventive and evidence-based medicine. This task force comprises primary care providers (i.e., internists, pediatricians, family physicians, gynecologists/obstetricians, nurses, and health behavior specialists). On July 30, 2013, the USPSTF released a draft recommendation statement posted for public comment on their Web site. The USPSTF further conducted a comprehensive review of the medical evidence for LDCT in the early detection of lung cancer including the NLST results and those from smaller randomized European trials with different eligibility criteria. The USPSTF also commissioned mathematical modeling studies to optimize information regarding the best patient ages to begin and end lung cancer screening, appropriate screening intervals, and the relative benefits and harms of different screening protocols.

On December 31, 2013, the USPSTF issued its final recommendation statement and also released a fact sheet to aid in the implementation of lung cancer–screening programs for high-risk individuals. The task force gave LDCT a "B" grade (the equivalent grade for screening mammography). The "B" grade indicates that there is *high certainty the net benefit is moderate* or there is *moderate certainty the net benefit is moderate to substantial* and that this particular service should be provided. Importantly, the Patient Protection and Affordable Care Act (ACA) requires private insurers to cover without co-pay all medical examinations or procedures receiving a grade "B" or higher from the USPSTF.

In particular, USPSTF recommended annual screening with LDCT in persons 55 to 80 years of age with the equivalent of a 30 pack-year of cigarette smoking who currently smoke or had quit within the past 15 years. They also recommended that screening should cease once the individual had not smoked for 15 years or developed health problems, significantly limiting their life expectancy, ability, or willingness to undergo curative lung resection surgery. The USPSTF evidence suggested implementing a screening program with these specific eligibility criteria would detect approximately one half of all lung cancers at an earlier, potentially resectable stage and could save as many as 20,000 lives each year in the United States.

The USPSTF also emphasized that the benefits of screening would be maximized when qualified health professionals do the following:

- Limit screening to high-risk persons.
- Accurately interpret the LDCT images.
- Strive to reduce false-positive studies in lieu of invasive procedures by additional imaging or short-term interval low-dose studies.
- Enroll current smokers into smoking cessation programs.

The ACR and the Radiological Society of North America (RSNA) immediately supported the USPSTF recommendations and developed standards to support lung cancer–screening programs across the country. The ACR in co-sponsorship with the Society of Thoracic Radiology (STR) subsequently released specific practice parameters for the performance and reporting of LDCT for the early detection of lung cancer in high-risk persons discussed later in this book.

3.7 Centers for Medicare & Medicaid Services

In February 2015, CMS issued its final decision to approve for reimbursement LDCT lung cancer screening for qualified Medicare beneficiaries. Those persons eligible for lung cancer screening under CMS guidelines are for the most part identical to those recommended by the USPSTF. Namely, current or former heavy smokers with the equivalent of a 30 pack-year of cigarette smoking that currently smoke or had quit smoking within the past 15 years. However, CMS did restrict the age of eligible persons with Medicare to 55 to 77 years as opposed to the 80 years recommended by the USPSTF. CMS also mandated that the primary health care provider or other qualified health care provider both *counsel* and *document* mutual participation in a shared decision-making visit prior to submitting a written order for lung cancer screening. The shared decision-making process must include a discussion regarding the benefits and potential harms of lung cancer screening, the need to adhere to annual screening and appropriate follow-up, reinforcing abstinence for former smokers, and cessation counseling or provision of resources for interested current smokers. These latter topics are discussed in further detail in Chapters 4 and 8.

Suggested Readings

[1] American College of Radiology. ACR Statement on USPSTF Draft Recommendation for CT Lung Cancer Screening. Available at: http://www.acr.org/About-Us/Media-Center/Press-Releases/2013-Press-Releases/20130729-ACR-Statement-on-USPSTF-Draft-Recommendation-for-CT-Lung-Cancer-Screening. Accessed March 1, 2017

[2] Yee KM. ACR, 40 Orgs call for Medicare Coverage of CT Lung Screening. Available at: http://www.auntminnie.com/index.aspx?sec = sup&sub = imc&pag = dis&ItemID = 106861. Accessed March 12, 2017

[3] American Cancer Society. Cancer Facts and Figures 2016. Available at: http://www.cancer.org/acs/groups/content/@epidemiologysurveilance/documents/document/acspc-036845.pdf. Accessed October 26, 2016

[4] American Cancer Society New Lung Cancer Screening Guidelines for Heavy Smokers. Available at: http://www.cancer.org/ cancer/news/new-lung-cancer-screening-guidelines-for-heavy- smokers

[5] American Lung Association. American Lung Association Provides Guidance on Lung Cancer Screening. Available at: http:// www.lung.org/lung-disease/lung-cancer/lung-cancer-screening- guidelines/

[6] Brett GZ. The value of lung cancer detection by six-monthly chest radiographs. Thorax. 1968; 23(4):414–420

[7] Dela Cruz CS, Tanoue LT, Matthay RA. Lung cancer: epidemiology, etiology, and prevention. Clin Chest Med. 2011; 32(4):605–644

[8] Detterbeck FC, Mazzone PJ, Naidich DP, Bach PB. Screening for lung cancer: Diagnosis and management of lung cancer, 3rd ed. American College of Chest Physicians evidence-based clinical practice guidelines. Chest. 2013; 143 5, Suppl:e78S–e92S

[9] Doria-Rose VP, Marcus PM, Szabo E, Tockman MS, Melamed MR, Prorok PC. Randomized controlled trials of the efficacy of lung cancer screening by sputum cytology revisited: a combined mortality analysis from the Johns Hopkins Lung Project and the Memorial Sloan-Kettering Lung Study. Cancer. 2009; 115(21):5007–5017

[10] Centers for Medicare & Medicaid Services. Factors CMS considers in referring topics to the Medicare Evidence Development & Coverage Advisory Committee. Available at: http://www.cms.gov/medicare-coverage-database/ details/medicare-coverage-document-details.aspx?MCDId = 10

[11] Fontana RS, Sanderson DR, Woolner LB, Taylor WF, Miller WE, Muhm JR. Lung cancer screening: the Mayo program. J Occup Med. 1986; 28(8):746–750

[12] Fontana RS. The Mayo Lung Project: a perspective. Cancer. 2000; 89(11) Suppl:2352–2355

[13] Friberg S, Mattson S. On the growth rates of human malignant tumors: implications for medical decision making. J Surg Oncol. 1997; 65(4):284–297

[14] Gill GW. Cytocentrifugation. In: Rosenthal D, ed. Cytopreparation: Principles & Practice. New York: Springer Science + Business; 2013: 44-71

[15] Shapiro S. History. In: Kramer BS, Gohagan JK, Prorok PC, eds. Cancer Screening: Theory and Practice. New York: Marcel Dekker, Inc.; 1999: 8-9

[16] Hayata Y, Funatsu H, Kato H, Saito Y, Sawamura K, Furose K. Results of lung cancer screening programs in Japan. Recent Results Cancer Res. 1982; 82:163–173

[17] Jaklitsch MT, Jacobson FL, Austin JH, et al. The American Association for Thoracic Surgery guidelines for lung cancer screening using low-dose computed tomography scans for lung cancer survivors and other high-risk groups. J Thorac Cardiovasc Surg. 2012; 144(1):33–38

[18] Kubík A, Polák J. Lung cancer detection. Results of a randomized prospective study in Czechoslovakia. Cancer. 1986; 57(12):2427–2437

[19] Lung Cancer Alliance. National Framework for Excellence in Lung Cancer Screening and Continuum of Care: Uniting the At-Risk Public with Responsible Medical Care Now. Available at: http://www.lungcanceralliance. org/get-information/am-i-at-risk/national-framework-for-lung-screening-excellence.html

[20] Lung Cancer Guidelines. Available at: http://www.asco.org/ guidelines/lung-cancer

[21] Manser RL, Irving LB, Byrnes G, Abramson MJ, Stone CA, Campbell DA. Screening for lung cancer: a systematic review and meta-analysis of controlled trials. Thorax. 2003; 58(9):784–789

[22] Manser RL, Irving LB, Stone C, Byrnes G, Abramson M, Campbell D. Screening for lung cancer. Cochrane Database Syst Rev. 2004(1):CD001991

[23] Medicare coverage determination process. Available at: http://www.cms.gov/Medicare/Coverage/ DeterminationProcess/

[24] Hansen HH, ed. Lung Cancer: Basic and Clinical Aspects. Boston, MA: Martinus Nijhoff Publishers; 1986

[25] Melamed MR, Flehinger BJ, Zaman MB, Heelan RT, Perchick WA, Martini N. Screening for early lung cancer. Results of the Memorial Sloan-Kettering study in New York. Chest. 1984; 86(1):44–53

[26] Moyer VA, U.S. Preventive Services Task Force. Screening for lung cancer: U.S. Preventive Services Task Force recommendation statement. Ann Intern Med. 2014; 160(5):330–338

[27] Muller FH. Tabakmissbrauch und Lungencarcinom. Z Krebsforsch. 1939; 49:57–85

[28] Nash FA, Morgan JM, Tomkins JG. South London Lung Cancer Study. BMJ. 1968; 2(5607):715–721

[29] National Comprehensive Cancer Network. Available at: https://www.nccn.org/store/login/login.aspx? ReturnURL = http://www. nccn.org /professionals/physician_gls/pdf/lung _screening.pdf

[30] National Cancer Institute (NCI) at the National Institutes of Health. National Lung Screening Trial (NLST). Available at: http://www.cancer.gov/clinicaltrials/noteworthy-trials/nlst/publications-from-nlst

[31] Aberle DR, Adams AM, Berg CD, et al. National Lung Screening Trial Research Team. Reduced lung-cancer mortality with low-dose computed tomographic screening. N Engl J Med. 2011; 365(5):395–409

[32] New Lung Cancer Guidelines Recommends Offering Screening to High-Risk Individuals. Available at: http://www .chestnet.org/ News/Press-Releases/2013/05/New-Lung-Cancer-Guidelines-Recommends-Establishment-of-Screening-Programs

[33] Oken MM, Hocking WG, Kvale PA, et al. PLCO Project Team. Screening by chest radiograph and lung cancer mortality: the Prostate, Lung, Colorectal, and Ovarian (PLCO) randomized trial. JAMA. 2011; 306(17):1865–1873

[34] Parker MS, Groves RC, Fowler AA, III, et al. Lung cancer screening with low-dose computed tomography: an analysis of the MEDCAC decision. J Thorac Imaging. 2015; 30(1):15–23

[35] Perlman EJ, Erozan YS, Howdon A. The role of the Saccomano technique in sputum cytopathologic diagnosis of lung cancer. Am J Clin Pathol. 1989; 91(1):57–60

[36] Proctor RN. The history of the discovery of the cigarette-lung cancer link: evidentiary traditions, corporate denial, global toll. Tob Control. 2012; 21(2):87–91

[37] RSNA Press Release. RSNA/ACR joint statement on lung cancer screening. Updated October 9, 2013. Available at: http://www2.rsna.org/timssnet/media/pressreleases/pr_target.cfm? ID = 693

[38] Saccomanno G, Archer VE, Auerbach O, Saunders RP, Brennan LM. Development of carcinoma of the lung as reflected in exfoliated cells. Cancer. 1974; 33(1):256–270

[39] Strauss GM, Gleason RE, Sugarbaker DJ. Screening for lung cancer. Another look; a different view. Chest. 1997; 111(3):754–768

[40] Tockman M. Survival and mortality from lung cancer in a screened population: the Johns Hopkins study. Chest. 1986; 89(Suppl):324S–325S

[41] US Preventive Services Task Forces. Available at: http://www.uspreventiveservicestaskforce.org

[42] US Preventive Services Task Force. Opportunities for public comment. Available at: http://www .uspreventiveservicestaskforce.org/tfcomment.htm

[43] Weiss W, Boucot KR, Cooper DA. The Philadelphia pulmonary neoplasm research project. Survival factors in bronchogenic carcinoma. JAMA. 1971; 216(13):2119–2123

[44] Wilde J. A 10 year follow-up of semi-annual screening for early detection of lung cancer in the Erfurt County, GDR. Eur Respir J. 1989; 2(7):656–662

4 Lung Cancer Screening Pros and Cons

Mark S. Parker

Summary

This chapter provides an in-depth discussion of the key elements of the shared decision-making process that must be fulfilled in order for providers, radiologists, and practices to not only appropriately screen, but also receive reimbursement for lung cancer–screening studies performed. The currently approved specific eligibility requirements for lung cancer screening are reviewed as well as the disparate risks and benefits of low-dose screening versus that of no screening are discussed. This chapter also highlights the false-positive, false-negative, and overdiagnosis rates associated with lung cancer screening. The radiation dose associated with LDCT (low-dose computed tomography) screening and the linear nonthreshold model of potential stochastic radiation effects is addressed. The cost-effectiveness of low-dose early detection lung cancer screening relative to that of other commonly employed screens such as colonoscopy and mammography are also examined.

Keywords: shared decision making, eligibility, false-positive rate, overdiagnosis, stochastic radiation effects, comorbidities, 1–800-QUITNOW, Cancer Intervention and Surveillance Modeling Network, www.shouldiscreen.com, American Academy of Family Physicians, COSMOS trial, ITALUNG RCT

4.1 The Shared Decision Making

Eligibility for potential lung cancer screening (LCS) requires that the intended individual(s) meet specifically defined criteria. Satisfaction of these criteria are required in accordance with the Medicare National Coverage Determination (NCD) for computed tomography (CT) LCS and must be met regardless of the individual's type of insurance coverage or even lack thereof.

The Centers for Medicare & Medicaid Services (CMS) determined there is sufficient evidence to add annual low-dose CT (LDCT) screening for the early detection of lung cancer for qualified beneficiaries as a preventative service benefit. Most third-party payers have now adopted the same stance. However, the LCS process first requires a shared decision-making visit. That is, an initial-face-to-face visit between the ordering primary health care provider (e.g., internist, family practitioner, pulmonologist, etc.) and the prospective screenee. During this shared decision-making visit, the primary health care provider must determine the individual's eligibility for screening, document their current and/or past cigarette use, discuss the benefits and potential harms of LDCT LCS, and counsel current cigarette smokers about cessation. This acquired information must also be documented in the individual's medical record. Primary health care providers and their patients should understand that LDCT LCS is not applicable to pipe, cigar, or marijuana smokers, but only former and current heavy cigarette smokers.

The primary health care provider must document in the individual's medical record or office notes the following information before the LDCT can be ordered or performed:

- Age: 55–77 years (CMS); 55–80 years (U.S. Preventive Services Task Forces [USPSTF]).
- Cigarette smoking history:
  - Current smoker: at least 1 pack per day (PPD) for 30 years or equivalent thereof.

○ Former smoker: at least 1 PPD for 30 years or equivalent thereof and has quit within the past 15 years.
- Asymptomatic: no current signs or symptoms of lung cancer (e.g., weight loss, new or changing cough, hemoptysis, etc.)
- Benefits and potential harms of LCS CT including (may use decision aids) the following:
  ○ False-positive rate.
  ○ Overdiagnosis.
  ○ Follow-up testing.
  ○ Total radiation exposure.
- Stress the importance of adherence to annual LDCT LCS.
- Reinforce the importance of abstinence if a former smoker and the importance of smoking cessation if a current smoker and, if appropriate, furnish information and resources to aid them in "kicking the habit" (1–800-QUITNOW; the National Cancer Institute [NCI]: 1–800–4-CANCER; the American Lung Association: 1–800-LUNG-USA; the American Heart Association: 1–800–242–872; Smokers' Helpline: 1–877–513–5333, etc.).
- Understand the concept that just because an individual can be screened does not necessarily mean they should be screened. Acknowledge the impact of a given individual's various comorbidities, their ability or willingness to undergo diagnosis, treatment, potential curative surgical resection, etc. (www.shouldiscreen.com).
- Written order for LDCT LCS.

4.2 Benefits and Potential Harms of Lung Cancer Screening

The American Academy of Family Physicians (AAFP) is one of the few medical societies that have not yet endorsed LDCT screening for the early detection of lung cancer. The AAFP contends that the USPSTF made unfounded and potentially costly recommendations based solely on the National Lung Screening Trial (NLST) results. The AAFP suggests the favorable NLST results may have been skewed because screening and treatment were conducted at major medical centers. Specifically, the AAFP contends the NLST was performed exclusively at those medical centers well known for their expertise in the imaging, diagnosis, and treatment of lung cancer and that the NLST results have not been replicated in community medical practices. The AAFP also argues that the long-term harms of radiation exposure from follow-up full-dose CT scans are unknown, and they are concerned about the number of patients who may undergo potentially unnecessary invasive bronchoscopy and surgical procedures.

In actuality, the USPSTF based its recommendations not only on the NLST results, but also included other U.S. and European studies, and sophisticated mathematical modeling exercises conducted by the NCI's Cancer Intervention and Surveillance Modeling Network (CISNET). Combining various models and the input in hundreds of diverse screening scenarios, the CISNET analysis revealed an average mortality reduction of 14% and further estimated that 50% of lung cancers would be detected at an early stage with LDCT screening. Their analysis suggests that nearly 500 lung cancer deaths could be prevented per 100,000 screened individuals. This mathematical model also revealed a benefit for screening even older persons from 74 to 80 years of age. Data from the Surveillance, Epidemiology, and End Results (SEER) program reveal that raising the upper age limit for screening to 80 years, as recommended by the USPSTF, would increase the number of detected lung cancers from about 40% among 55- to 74-year-olds to about 60% among 55- to 80-year-olds. In September 2014, a new analysis of data from the NLST was published concluding LDCT LCS is even more effective in older Medicare-aged individuals than in younger persons. Pinsky and colleagues divided the NLST participants into two groups: older current and former heavy smokers aged 65 to 74 years and younger persons aged 55 to 64 years with similar smoking histories. The researchers found a higher prevalence of lung cancer in the older Medicare-aged group (1.5 vs. 0.7%) and that LDCT screening also had a higher positive predictive value in these latter Medicare-eligible persons (4.9 vs. 3.0%; p <0.001) necessitating a fewer number of screens to prevent one lung cancer death (245 vs. 364 screens).

There is a misconception that all NLST participants were imaged and treated at major academic medical centers and that the positive results of the NLST are unlikely to be reproducible in community-based practices. In reality, about 25% of participating NLST medical centers were not tertiary care academic medical centers. To the best of our knowledge, no definitive clinical evidence has been published to support the concern that potential risks of LCS will be accentuated in community medical practices. Numerous community databases have shown no statistically significant difference between academic and community-based programs.

Lung cancer is often an insidious disease, producing minimal or no clinical symptoms until it is far advanced and no longer curable by surgical resection. Most patients already have locally advanced or metastatic disease at their first clinical presentation. Only 15 to 25% of patients have potentially resectable, early- stage disease confined to the chest at presentation. If a lung cancer is not resectable when it is first discovered, most affected patients will die within the next 9 months. Despite surgical and chemoradiation therapy advances, the 5-year survival rate for all newly diagnosed lung cancers of all stages remains a dismal 16 to 17% (~ 1 in 7). That is the harm of not screening for lung cancer. Alternatively, in the NLST, 412 patients (85%) were diagnosed with clinical stage I lung cancer. The estimated 10-year survival rate in this subgroup is 88%. Among 302 participants with clinical stage I cancer who underwent surgical resection within 1 month after diagnosis, the survival rate was 92%. That is the disparate benefit of LDCT LCS.

4.3 False-Negative Rate

Currently no gold standard exists for assessing true-negative screening results on LDCT. The sensitivity is usually determined by the detection of a lung cancer within 1 year of the initial screening study on a follow-up LDCT screen. As of this writing, six studies have reported the sensitivity of LDCT for detecting lung cancer ranging from 80 to 100% (most often > 90%), and a resultant false-negative rate of 0 to 20%. These values are contrasted with the false-negative rates of both screening mammography and flexible sigmoidoscopy in ▶ Table 4.1. The data suggest screening with LDCT for the early

Table 4.1 False-negative rate screening exam comparisons

Screening test	False (−) rate (%)
LDCT lung cancer screening	0–20
Mammography	20
Flexible sigmoidoscopy	48
Abbreviation: LDCT, low-dose computed tomography.	

detection of lung cancer is more efficacious than screening mammography or flexible sigmoidoscopy.

4.4 False-Positive Rate

LCS with LDCT, like other clinically relied upon screens, may be associated with false-positive results, that is, suggesting the presence of cancer when indeed there is not. In the NLST, a screen was deemed "positive" when a noncalcified nodule measuring at least 4 mm in diameter was detected. Across the baseline and two subsequent annual rounds of screens, 96% of the positive LDCT screens and 95% of the chest X-ray screens were falsely positive. However, we would like to emphasize that simply detecting a lung nodule does not necessarily commit that individual to an invasive procedure. The presence of a nodule does not dictate that that particular individual must have a biopsy. LDCT is an imaging-based and not tissue-based screening program. Ninety-six percent of false-positive findings are sorted out with short-term, 3- to 6-month repeat LDCT imaging (▶ Fig. 4.1), not invasive procedures, biopsy or surgery, but rather through imaging alone. The American College of Radiology (ACR) has developed a "Lung CT Screening Reporting and Data System" (Lung-RADS) for specific reporting, follow-up, and management of both negative and positive LDCT screens, which is discussed further in Chapter 6. Recently, the ACR increased the size threshold for a "positive" screen from the 4-mm diameter used in NLST to a 6-mm diameter on the basis of a large amount of supporting data. The ACR also increased the dimension for a positive ground glass nodule to greater than 20 mm. It is anticipated that this simple change in an "actionable nodule" diameter will substantially reduce the number of false-positive studies compared with NLST. The ACR Lung-RADS classification scheme (Chapter 6) for LCS, similar to the "Bi-RADs" system for screening mammography, is expected to markedly reduce the workup of positive studies and further stratify the pertinent imaging findings. By applying the Lung-RADS system, it is estimated that only 1 in 10 persons with a positive LDCT screen may require a biopsy. Comparing the false-positive rates and guidelines used for the management of positive study results, and the number of lives saved per screening, once again, LDCT is a more efficacious screen than the already accepted and widely utilized screening mammography and flexible sigmoidoscopy as shown in ▶ Table 4.2.

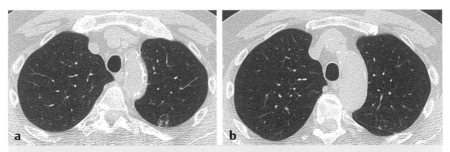

Fig. 4.1 A 62-year-old man with a false-positive baseline lung cancer screening computed tomography (CT) sorted out via short-term repeat low-dose computed tomography (LDCT). **(a)** Baseline LDCT shows a 16-mm part-solid nodule in the peripheral apical posterior segment of the left upper lobe bordering the oblique fissure. **(b)** Follow-up LDCT 3 months following a short course of steroids shows near complete resolution of the lesion of concern. Diagnosis: presumed focus of organizing pneumonia.

Table 4.2 False-positive rates of other accepted screens versus low-dose computed tomography (LDCT)

Screening test	False (+) results (%)	Cancer deaths prevented
LDCT lung cancer screening	96	1 per 320 screens
Mammography	50–60	1 per 1,905 screens
Flexible sigmoidoscopy	30.3 (men)/19.3 (women)	1 per 871 screens

4.5 Overdiagnosis Rate

Overdiagnosis may be considered an extreme form of length-time bias. This concept is also sometimes referred to as "pseudo-disease." Although such lesions fulfill the histologic criteria for neoplasia, not all lung cancers are created equal. There is significant biologic variability in the behavior of certain types of lung cancers. Some particular tumors tend to grow so slowly that they will not cause harm to or kill the affected individual (▶ Fig. 4.2). These are lung cancers the affected person may die with rather than die from, succumbing to other comorbid factors first (e.g., heart disease and stroke).

Overdiagnosis is not unique to LDCT screening but rather intrinsic to cancer screening in general. For example, screening mammograms can detect breast cancers and cases of ductal carcinoma in situ (DCIS). This noninvasive tumor does indeed require appropriate treatment. However, screening mammography may also find cancers and

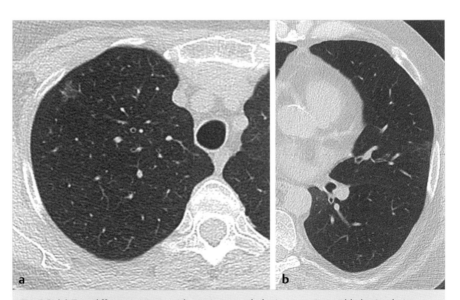

Fig. 4.2 (a) Two different patients with varying morphologic appearing and behaving lesions detected on low-dose computed tomography (LDCT) that may or may not ever cause harm to the patient (potential overdiagnosis). A 64-year-old woman with a 10 × 11 mm ground glass opacity detected in the peripheral anterior segment of the right upper lobe. Diagnosis: atypical adenomatous hyperplasia. A 63-year-old man with a 10-mm part-solid lung nodule detected in the lingula. **(b)** The solid component measured 2 mm. Diagnosis: minimally invasive adenocarcinoma.

other cases of DCIS that will never cause symptoms or threaten the woman's life, thereby resulting in an "overdiagnosis" of breast cancer. Most often, we cannot clinically distinguish those cancers and cases of DCIS that do and do not require treatment and thus all detected cancers are similarly treated. Overdiagnosis then results in "overtreatment," exposing these particular women to unnecessary additional imaging, biopsy, surgery, and potentially chemotherapy and radiation therapy.

Analogously, in the NLST, investigators found that about 18% or approximately one in five cancers detected at LDCT were likely indolent. Such lung cancers are so slow growing that they are unlikely to ever cause symptoms or harm the patient. But, like some cases of DCIS, there are no easy radiologic or clinical means at this time to determine which of these lesions may require aggressive management and which ones will not. The number of cases of overdiagnosis found among the 320 NLST participants who would need to be screened to prevent one death from lung cancer was 1.38. The NLST investigators stressed that the overdiagnosis rate is likely to diminish as further experience is gained and that this estimate is likely an upper limit of the potential overdiagnosis rate for LDCT. Supporting their hypothesis, the USPSTF modeling studies estimate that only 10 to 12% of screen-detected lung cancer cases would not otherwise be detected in a patient's lifetime.

4.6 Radiation Exposure

LCS with LDCT uses ionizing radiation. Clinical concerns have been raised regarding the stochastic risks of radiation-induced carcinogenesis from diagnostic and screening CTs. These concerns and purported potential adverse stochastic effects of ionizing radiation are based on modeling studies from the radiation exposure incurred by the 1945 atomic bomb survivors in Hiroshima and Nagasaki and/or nuclear power plant accidents applying the linear nonthreshold (LNT) theory. This theory postulates that any and all radiation exposure is harmful and carcinogenic. The validity of the LNT model has been called into question, but it remains debated by radiation physicists and other experts. Equally important, the LNT model was originally developed as a protection guideline for "occupationally" exposed individuals. The LNT was not developed as an attempt to predict potential increased stochastic effects or possible cancer deaths in persons exposed to "medical doses of ionizing radiation."

The risk of developing cancer from LDCT LCS is likely very small. In fact, the risk is estimated to be smaller than that of a smoker developing lung cancer in the absence of screening. One model reported by Marshall et al predicts an excess lifetime risk of only 0.85% (95% confidence interval [CI]: 0.28–2.2%) for a 50-year-old female smoker receiving 25 annual LDCT scans. This compares to a 17% risk of her developing lung cancer in her lifetime without screening. de González et al estimated the cumulative risk of excess death from lung cancer from LDCT screens of 50-year-old smokers to be about 2 per 10,000 men and about 5 per 10,000 women screened. These investigators also predicted the possibility of about 3 cases of breast cancer per 10,000 women screened. However, LCS would likely result in 30 fewer deaths per 10,000 individuals screened. Italian Lung Cancer Screening Trial (ITALUNG) randomized clinical trial (RCT) drew similar conclusions, predicting about 1.1 excess death per 10,000 persons screened compared to about 15 to 100 lives saved per 10,000 women and men screened. Rampinelli et al retrospectively analyzed data from the 10-year nonrandomized CT for LCS (COSMOS [Continuous Observation of Smoking Subjects]) trial that scanned asymptomatic individuals at increased risk for lung cancer. Specifically, those persons over 50 years of age with at least a 20-pack-year history of tobacco abuse. In all, 5,203 asymptomatic high risk-persons (3,439 men and 1,764 women) underwent LDCT screens for 10 consecutive years in Milan, Italy, between 2004 and 2015. Rampinelli and colleagues matched these individuals by age, sex, weight, and body habitus to 11 gender-specific phantoms to create size-specific organ doses and calculated the potential cancer risks for both men and women and organ system based on the National Research Council's 2006 BEIR VII report. Over this 10 year study period, these 5,203 persons received 42,228 LDCT scans. The mean cumulative radiation dose following the 10th year of screening was 9.3 mSv for men and 13.0 mSv for women. They calculated that the lifetime attributable risk of lung cancer following 10 years of LDCT screens ranged from 1.4 to 5.5 cases per 10,000 men and for other major cancers 2.6 to 8.1 per 10,000 persons screened. These investigators further deducted that 10 years of LDCT screening could possibly induce 1.5 lung cancers and 2.4 other major cancers corresponding to an additional risk of induced cancers of 0.05% compared with 259 lung cancers that were diagnosed during the 10-year screening period. Rampinelli et al concluded that after 10 years of LDCT screening 1 theoretically induced major cancer might be expected for every 108 lung cancers detected through the screening process. A key point to remember is that the risk of radiation-induced carcinogenesis decreases with increasing age. Thus, the radiation risk-to-benefit ratio of LCS with LDCT is more than acceptable in this otherwise older high-risk population. Once again, the current body of literature supports that more high-risk persons are likely to die from undetected lung cancers in the absence of a screening program than are likely to develop lung or other major cancers from the process of LDCT screening.

Diagnostic radiologists are well aware of these clinical concerns. It should be emphasized to all nonradiologists and potential screened persons that radiologists receive dedicated training in radiation safety and in dose-saving techniques in accordance with the "as low as reasonably achievable" (ALARA) principle—that is, performing diagnostic imaging studies including screens with those doses of ionizing radiation that are ALARA to provide a diagnostic quality examination. LDCT LCS and the imaging guidelines developed by the ACR for LCS epitomize the ALARA principle. The CT radiation dose is determined by patient body habitus, tube current, tube voltage, various filters, and scan length (Z-axis). In LDCT LCS studies, radiologists most commonly limit the radiation dose by adjusting the tube current (mA) based upon the scanned person's weight. Since image quality is inversely proportional to the square root of the dose, some may find the LDCT images somewhat more "noisy" than standard dose chest CT images. The increased noise is especially noticeable through the thoracic inlet and the upper abdomen. Although noisier, rest assured the screening studies are still of diagnostic quality because of the inherently high contrast between air-filled lung tissue and soft-tissue lung nodules. Radiologists are able to reduce the mean effective dose from an average of 8 mSv (standard chest CT) to approximately 1.5 mSv for most standard screening studies without sacrificing image quality or scan resolution. The total accumulative lifetime radiation dose can be further limited by encouraging referral services and radiologists to strictly adhere to the Lung-RADS management guidelines for interim or follow-up screens.

4.7 Cost-Effectiveness Relative to Other Screening Exams

Many concerns have been raised regarding whether the health care system can afford the projected costs of a national LCS program. Joshua A. Roth, PhD, MHA, a postdoctoral research fellow at the Fred Hutchinson Cancer Research Center in Seattle, WA, showed that adding LDCT screening to the Medicare program could result in the diagnosis of about 54,900 earlier-stage and more treatable lung cancers over a 5-year period. At the 2014 Annual Meeting of the American Society of Clinical Oncology, Dr. Roth postulated that about $5.6 billion would be spent on an estimated 11.2 million additional LDCT scans over the next 5 years. Approximately $1.1 billion would be spent on diagnostic workups, and $2.6 billion would be spent on cancer care, for a total cost of $9.3 billion to Medicare. Thus, it is imperative that Medicare and other third-party payer systems prepare not only for the increased demand for LDCT imaging, but also for the treatment of early-stage lung cancers. To put this total 5-year expenditure into perspective, the costs would amount to only a $3.00/month increase in premiums per Medicare member. A study conducted by the actuarial firm Milliman also found that implementing the screening recommendations proposed by the USPSTF would be highly cost-effective. Pyenson and colleagues further found that LDCT screening in high-risk Medicare-aged persons was more cost-effective than screening for cervical and breast cancer and was comparable to that of colorectal cancer screening. Applying the USPSTF guidelines, the researchers determined that 4.9 million Medicare beneficiaries would be eligible for screening in 2014. If all 4.9 million beneficiaries were screened and treated consistently beginning at age 55 years, approximately 358,000 additional people with current or prior lung cancer would still be alive. Pyenson et al estimated that the total cost of a life-year saved with LDCT is $18,452 with an estimated average annual cost of $241 per person screened.

Suggested Readings

[1] Centers for Medicare & Medicaid Services. Decision Memo for Screening for Lung Cancer with Low Dose Computed Tomography (LDCT) (CAG-00439N). Available online at: https://www.cms.gov/medicare-coverage-database/details/nca-decision-memo.aspx?NCAId=274

[2] American College of Radiology. CT Lung Cancer Screening Shared Decision Making Visit Requirements. Available at: https://www.acr.org/~/media/ACR/Documents/PDF/QualitySafety/NRDR/Lung-Cancer-Screening-Practice-Registry/Shared-Decision-Making-Tools/shared_decision_making_memo.pdf?la=en

[3] National Cancer Institute. Fact Sheets and Brochures. Available at: http://surveillance.cancer.gov/publications/factsheets/

[4] National Cancer Institute. The Cancer Intervention and Surveillance Modeling Network (CISNET). Available at: http://surveillance.cancer.gov/publications/factsheets/CISNET_Fact_Sheet.pdf

[5] U.S. Preventive Services. Available at: http://www.uspreventiveservicestaskforce.org/uspstf13/lungcan/lungcanmodeling.pdf

[6] U.S. Preventive Services. Available at: http://www.uspreventiveservicestaskforce.org/uspstf13/lungcan/lungcanfact.pdf

[7] Alvarado M, Ozanne E, Esserman L. Overdiagnosis and overtreatment of breast cancer. Am Soc Clin Oncol Educ Book. 2012:e40–e45

[8] American Academy of Family Physicians. Summary of Recommendations for Clinical Preventive Services-Lung Cancer. Available at: http://www.aafp.org/dam/AAFP/documents/patient_care/clinical_recommendations/cps-recommendations.pdf

[9] American Cancer Society. Cancer Facts and Figures 2015. Available at: http://www.cancer.org/acs/groups/content/@epidemiologysurveilance/documents/document/acspc-036845.pdf

[10] de González AB, Kim KP, Berg CD. Low-dose lung computed tomography screening before age 55: estimates of the mortality reduction required to outweigh the radiation-induced cancer risk. J Med Screen. 2008; 15 (3):153–158

[11] de González AB, Darby S. Risk of cancer from diagnostic X-rays: estimates for the UK and 14 other countries. Lancet. 2004; 363(9406):345–351

[12] Boone JM, Hendee WR, McNitt-Gray MF, Seltzer SE. Radiation exposure from CT scans: how to close our knowledge gaps, monitor and safeguard exposure–proceedings and recommendations of the Radiation Dose Summit, sponsored by NIBIB, February 24–25, 2011. Radiology. 2012; 265(2):544–554

[13] Brenner DJ. Radiation risks potentially associated with low-dose CT screening of adult smokers for lung cancer. Radiology. 2004; 231(2):440–445

[14] Calabrese EJ. The road to linearity: why linearity at low doses became the basis for carcinogen risk assessment. Arch Toxicol. 2009; 83(3):203–225

[15] Advisory Board Company. Congress Agrees: Medicare Should Cover Lung Cancer Screening. Available at: http://www.advisory.com/research/imaging-performance-partnership/the-reading-room/2014/06/congress-agrees-medicare-should-cover-lung-cancer-screening

[16] Croswell JM, Kramer BS, Kreimer AR, et al. Cumulative incidence of false-positive results in repeated, multimodal cancer screening. Ann Fam Med. 2009; 7(3):212–222

[17] Lung Cancer Screening Would Cost Medicare CT. $9 Billion. Available at: http://www.medscape.com/viewarticle/825235#1

[18] Grannis FW Jr. CT Lung Screening Meeting: A Travesty of Public Health Policy. Available at: http://www.auntminnie.com/index.aspx?sec=sup&sub=imc&pag=dis&ItemID=107339&wf=1

[19] de Koning HJ, Meza R, Plevritis SK, et al. Benefits and harms of computed tomography lung cancer screening strategies: a comparative modeling study for the U.S. Preventive Services Task Force. Ann Intern Med. 2014; 160(5):311–320

[20] Ellis PM, Vandermeer R. Delays in the diagnosis of lung cancer. J Thorac Dis. 2011; 3(3):183–188

[21] Elmore JG, Barton MB, Moceri VM, Polk S, Arena PJ, Fletcher SW. Ten-year risk of false positive screening mammograms and clinical breast examinations. N Engl J Med. 1998; 338(16):1089–1096

[22] Gøtzsche PC, Jørgensen KJ. Screening for breast cancer with mammography. Cochrane Database Syst Rev. 2013; 6(6):CD001877

[23] Henschke CI, Yankelevitz DF, Libby DM, Pasmantier MW, Smith JP, Miettinen OS, International Early Lung Cancer Action Program Investigators. Survival of patients with stage I lung cancer detected on CT screening. N Engl J Med. 2006; 355(17):1763–1771

[24] Herzog P, Rieger CT. Risk of cancer from diagnostic X-rays. Lancet. 2004; 363(9406):340–341

[25] Hubbard RA, Kerlikowske K, Flowers CI, Yankaskas BC, Zhu W, Miglioretti DL. Cumulative probability of false-positive recall or biopsy recommendation after 10 years of screening mammography: a cohort study. Ann Intern Med. 2011; 155(8):481–492

[26] Kazerooni EA, Austin JHM, Black WC, et al. American College of Radiology, Society of Thoracic Radiology. ACR-STR practice parameter for the performance and reporting of lung cancer screening thoracic computed tomography (CT): 2014 (Resolution 4). J Thorac Imaging. 2014; 29(5):310–316

[27] Kubo T, Lin P-JP, Stiller W, et al. Radiation dose reduction in chest CT: a review. AJR Am J Roentgenol. 2008; 190(2):335–343

[28] Lung CT Screening Reporting and Data System (Lung-RADS). Available at: http://www.acr.org/Quality-Safety/Resources/LungRADS

[29] Marshall HM, Bowman RV, Yang IA, Fong KM, Berg CD. Screening for lung cancer with low-dose computed tomography: a review of current status. J Thorac Dis. 2013; 5 Suppl 5:S524–S539

[30] Marshall H, Smith I, Keir B, et al. Radiation dose during lung cancer screening with low-dose computed tomography: how low is low dose? J Thorac Oncol. 2010; 363:345–351

[31] Mascalchi M, Mazzoni LN, Falchini M, et al. Dose exposure in the ITALUNG trial of lung cancer screening with low-dose CT. Br J Radiol. 2012; 85(1016):1134–1139

[32] Mascalchi M, Belli G, Zappa M, et al. Risk-benefit analysis of X-ray exposure associated with lung cancer screening in the Italung-CT trial. AJR Am J Roentgenol. 2006; 187(2):421–429

[33] Barnes E. Medicare Panel Raises Doubts about CT Lung Cancer Screening. Available at: http://www.auntminnie.com/index.aspx?sec=sup&sub=cto&pag=dis&ItemID=107278&wf=1

[34] McMahon PM, Hazelton WD, Kimmel M, Clarke LD. Chapter 13: CISNET lung models: comparison of model assumptions and model structures. Risk Anal. 2012; 32 Suppl 1:S166–S178

[35] Menezes RJ, Roberts HC, Paul NS, et al. Lung cancer screening using low-dose computed tomography in at-risk individuals: the Toronto experience. Lung Cancer. 2010; 67(2):177–183

[36] Centers for Medicare & Medicaid Services. Meeting minutes of the Centers for Medicare and Medicaid Services: Medicare Evidence Development & Coverage Advisory Committee. Available at: http://www.cms.gov/Regulations-and-Guidance/Guidance/FACA/downloads/id68d.pdf

[37] Meza R, ten Haaf K, Kong CY, et al. Comparative analysis of 5 lung cancer natural history and screening models that reproduce outcomes of the NLST and PLCO trials. Cancer. 2014; 120(11):1713–1724

[38] Moyer VA, U.S. Preventive Services Task Force. Screening for lung cancer: U.S. Preventive Services Task Force recommendation statement. Ann Intern Med. 2014; 160(5):330–338

[39] Aberle DR, Adams AM, Berg CD, et al. National Lung Screening Trial Research Team. Reduced lung-cancer mortality with low-dose computed tomographic screening. N Engl J Med. 2011; 365(5):395–409

[40] National Cancer Institute (NCI) at the National Institutes of Health. National Lung Screening Trial (NLST). Available at: http://www.cancer.gov/clinicaltrials/noteworthy-trials/nlst/publications-from-nlst

[41] National Cancer Institute. Cancer Intervention and Surveillance Modeling Network: Lung Cancer Modeling. Available at: http://cisnet.cancer.gov/lung

[42] National Cancer Institute Fact Sheet. Mammograms. Available at: http://www.cancer.gov/cancertopics/factsheet/detection/mammograms

[43] Barnes E. NLST Data Show Lung Cancer Screening is Ready. Available at: http://www.auntminnie.com/index.aspx?sec=sup&sub=cto&pag=dis&ItemID=106990

[44] Parker MS, Groves RC, Fowler AA, III, et al. Lung cancer screening with low-dose computed tomography: an analysis of the MEDCAC decision. J Thorac Imaging. 2015; 30(1):15–23

[45] Patz EF, Jr, Pinsky P, Gatsonis C, et al. NLST Overdiagnosis Manuscript Writing Team. Overdiagnosis in low-dose computed tomography screening for lung cancer. JAMA Intern Med. 2014; 174(2):269–274

[46] Pinsky PF, Berg CD. Applying the National Lung Screening Trial eligibility criteria to the US population: what percent of the population and of incident lung cancers would be covered? J Med Screen. 2012; 19(3):154–156

[47] Pinsky PF, Gierada DS, Hocking W, et al. National Lung Screening Trial findings by age: Medicare-eligible versus under-65 population. Ann Intern Med. 2014; 161(9):627–633

[48] Preston RJ. Update on linear non-threshold dose-response model and implications for diagnostic radiology procedures. Health Phys. 2008; 95(5):541–546

[49] Pyenson BS, Henschke CI, Yankelevitz DF, Yip R, Dec E. Offering lung cancer screening to high-risk Medicare beneficiaries saves lives and is cost-effective: an actuarial analysis. Am Health Drug Benefits. 2014; 7(5):272–282

[50] Rampinelli C, De Marco P, Origgi D, et al. Exposure to low dose computed tomography for lung cancer screening and risk of cancer: secondary analysis of trial data and risk-benefit analysis. BMJ. 2017; 356:j347

[51] Roth JA, Sullivan SD, Ravelo A, et al. Low-dose computed tomography lung cancer screening in the Medicare program: projected clinical, resource, and budget impact. J Clin Oncol. 2014; 32 15, Suppl:6501

[52] Schoen RE, Pinsky PF, Weissfeld JL, et al. Colorectal cancers not detected by screening flexible sigmoidoscopy in the Prostate, Lung, Colorectal, and Ovarian Cancer Screening Trial. Gastrointest Endosc. 2012; 75(3):612–620

[53] Swensen SJ, Jett JR, Hartman TE, et al. CT screening for lung cancer: five-year prospective experience. Radiology. 2005; 235(1):259–265

[54] Toyoda Y, Nakayama T, Kusunoki Y, Iso H, Suzuki T. Sensitivity and specificity of lung cancer screening using chest low-dose computed tomography. Br J Cancer. 2008; 98(10):1602–1607

[55] Tsushima K, Sone S, Hanaoka T, Kubo K. Radiological diagnosis of small pulmonary nodules detected on low-dose screening computed tomography. Respirology. 2008; 13(6):817–824

[56] USPSTF. Screen High-Risk Smokers for Lung Cancer. Available at: http://www.medpagetoday.com/HematologyOncology/LungCancer/40733

[57] van Klaveren RJ, Oudkerk M, Prokop M, et al. Management of lung nodules detected by volume CT scanning. N Engl J Med. 2009; 361(23):2221–2229

[58] Veronesi G, Bellomi M, Mulshine JL, et al. Lung cancer screening with low-dose computed tomography: a non-invasive diagnostic protocol for baseline lung nodules. Lung Cancer. 2008; 61(3):340–349

[59] Veronesi G, Bellomi M, Scanagatta P, et al. Difficulties encountered managing nodules detected during a computed tomography lung cancer screening program. J Thorac Cardiovasc Surg. 2008; 136(3):611–617

5 Variable Imaging Presentations of Lung Cancer

Mark S. Parker

Summary

This chapter reviews the most common location and imaging characteristics of missed lung cancers as well as the variable imaging presentations of lung cancers. The newly revised classification system for adenocarcinoma of the lung is also discussed. Illustrative examples of adenocarcinoma in situ, minimally invasive adenocarcinoma, and invasive adenocarcinoma are provided. The concept of malignancy rate based on lesion morphology and doubling times is also presented.

Keywords: missed lung cancers, adenocarcinoma, classification, atypical adenomatous hyperplasia, minimally invasive adenocarcinoma, adenocarcinoma in situ, invasive adenocarcinoma, lepidic, mucinous, solid, subsolid, ground glass, doubling time

5.1 Introduction

On conventional chest radiography, the variable manifestations of lung cancer may be broadly characterized as indirect or direct. Indirect radiographic manifestations include atelectasis, often related to an endobronchial lesion or extrinsic compression of the airway by adjacent lymphadenopathy and nonresolving pneumonia-airspace disease. Direct radiographic manifestations of lung cancer may include a nodule(s) (< 3.0 cm diameter), mass (≥ 3.0 cm diameter), and parenchymal consolidation (▶ Table 5.1).

5.2 Location and Imaging Characteristic of Missed Lung Cancers

As stressed earlier, conventional radiography is not the optimal screening tool for the early detection of lung cancer. Austin et al reported the vast majority of missed bronchogenic cancers on retrospective review occur in an upper lobe (81%) (3 upper lobe: 2 lower lobe), and in the right upper lobe in particular (56%) (3 RUL: 2 LUL). More missed lung cancers occurred in women (67%) than in men (33%). Other problematic radiographic regions where missed lung cancers occurred included the perihilar and paraspinal regions (▶ Fig. 5.1). The mean diameter of the missed lung cancer was 1.6 ± 0.8 cm (range: 0.6–3.4 cm). Shah et al revisited this topic in 2003 and again found that most missed potentially resectable primary lung cancers were located in the upper

Table 5.1 Variable radiographic manifestations of lung cancer

Indirect signs	Direct signs
Atelectasis	Nodule
Nonresolving pneumonia-airspace disease	Mass
	Focal consolidation

33

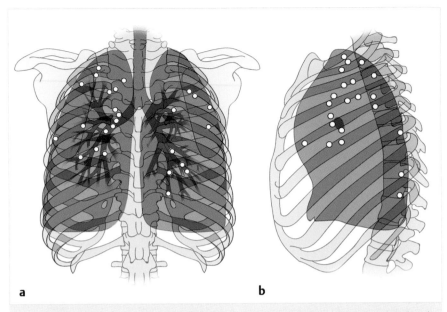

a   b

Fig. 5.1 **(a)** Most frequent location of missed primary lung cancers on posteroanterior (PA) and **(b)** lateral chest X-ray. (Adapted with permission of Austin JH, Romney BM, Goldsmith LS. Missed bronchogenic carcinoma: radiographic findings in 27 patients with a potentially resectable lesion evident in retrospect. Radiology. 1992;182(1):115–122.)

lobes (right: 45%; left: 28%; total: 72%), especially the apical and posterior segments or subsegments (60%). The clavicle obscured visualization of 22% of the missed cancers. The missed cancers had a median diameter of 1.9 cm. The high percentage (54–90%) and large average size (1.3–1.6 cm) of missed primary lung cancers on conventional chest radiographs have been reported in numerous additional studies. Potential contributing causes for failed radiographic detection include obscuration of the lesion from superimposed intrathoracic and extrathoracic structures such as the ribs, clavicles, hilar vessels, and the heart.

In 2002, Li et al reported 83 primary lung cancers were found during an annual low-dose computed tomography (LDCT) screen and confirmed at either biopsy or surgery. Thirty-two (38.6%) of these lung cancers were missed on 39 initial CT scans: 23 scans due to detection errors and 16 scans from interpretation errors. All of the missed lung cancers were intrapulmonary. Of these missed cancers, 88% were stage IA. All detection error cases involved adenocarcinomas. Eighty-five percent were well-differentiated lesions and 55% were in nonsmoking women. The mean size of missed cancers in this patient population was 9.8 mm. The mean size of missed lung cancers due to interpretation error was 15.9 mm. Ninety-one percent of the missed nodules in the detection error group were ground glass. In the detection error group, 83% of the missed lung cancers overlapped with or were obscured by similar-appearing adjacent normal structures such as pulmonary vessels. In all, 87.5% of CT scans with interpretation errors were associated with a background of concomitant complex disease. Most missed cancers tended to be central or endobronchial, adjacent to scars or vessels and of low attenuation.

On LDCT, lung cancers may have a variable appearance. Lesions may appear as well-defined, solid noncalcified nodules, subsolid pure ground-glass, and as part-solid nodules. Additional morphologic features may include lobulation, concave notching, desmoplasia, pleural retraction, internal lucencies, and pericystic nodularity. These varying morphologic appearances will be illustrated in the remainder of this textbook.

5.3 Revised Adenocarcinoma Classification

Non–small cell lung cancers (NSCLC) account for about 85% of all newly diagnosed lung cancers. Adenocarcinoma is the most common variety. The prevalence of adenocarcinoma is increasing and it presents more frequently in asymptomatic women, and often in nonsmokers. Recently, the International Association for the Study of Lung Cancer/ American Thoracic Society/European Respiratory Society (IASLC/ATS/ERS) introduced new terminology and diagnostic criteria to better reflect our understanding of the heterogeneous pathology, imaging features, and clinical behavior of peripheral lung adenocarcinomas (formerly known as bronchioloalveolar cell carcinoma). The new classification system clearly distinguishes between preinvasive, minimally invasive, and frankly invasive lung lesions (▶ Table 5.2).

The imaging spectrum of these precancerous and cancerous lesions ranges from pure ground-glass nodules to part-solid nodules to solid nodules and masses (▶ Fig. 5.2). A pure ground-glass nodule manifests as a focal area of increased attenuation that does not obscure visualization of the underlying lung parenchyma (e.g., bronchovascular bundles; ▶ Fig. 5.3a; ▶ Fig. 5.4). A subsolid nodule is an opacity that is less dense than solid and is further subdivided into part solid and pure ground glass (▶ Fig. 5.2). A part-solid nodule contains both solid high-attenuation elements and ground glass (▶ Fig. 5.5). A solid nodule manifests as a focal region of increased attenuation through which normal bronchovascular structures cannot be seen or are completely obscured (▶ Fig. 5.6).

Noguchi et al demonstrated that those patients with ground-glass nodular opacities identified on screening LDCT have a better prognosis than patients with solid nodules.

Table 5.2 New classification schema for lung adenocarcinoma (formerly bronchioloalveolar cell carcinoma)

Pre-invasive lesions	Minimally invasive lesions	Invasive adenocarcinoma	Invasive adenocarcinoma variants
Atypical adenomatous hyperplasia (AAH)	Minimally invasive adenocarcinomas (MIA; e.g., mucinous, nonmucinous, or mixed)	Acinar predominant	Invasive mucinous adenocarcinoma
Adenocarcinoma in situ (AIS; e.g., mucinous, nonmucinous, or mixed)		Papillary predominant	Colloid, fetal, and enteric
		Micropapillary predominant	
		Solid predominant with mucin production	
		Lepidic predominant adenocarcinoma	

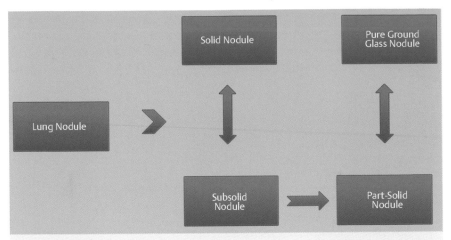

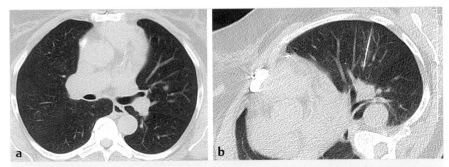

Fig. 5.2 Characterization of lung nodules on low-dose computed tomography (LDCT) using the new classification schema.

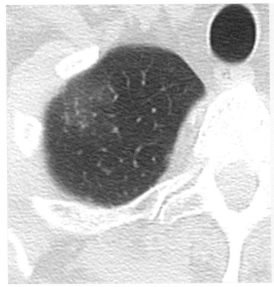

a b

Fig. 5.3 **(a)** Low-dose computed tomography (LDCT) scan of an asymptomatic woman smoker reveals a 5-mm pure ground-glass lesion in the lingula. Imaging features are consistent with atypical adenomatous hyperplasia. **(b)** The diagnosis was subsequently proven at biopsy.

Fig. 5.4 Low-dose computed tomography (LDCT) screening examination shows a 25-mm pure ground-glass opacity in the anterior segment of the right upper lobe. Diagnosis: adenocarcinoma in situ (AIS).

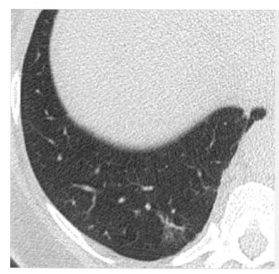

Fig. 5.5 Low-dose computed tomography (LDCT) screening examination shows a part-solid nodule with a small central component measuring less than 5 mm characteristic of minimally invasive adenocarcinoma (MIA) in the posterior basal segment of the right lower lobe

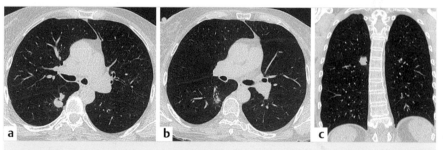

Fig. 5.6 (a,b) Selected axial and (c) coronal low-dose computed tomography (LDCT) images of a 60-year-old woman with a 40-pack-year history of tobacco abuse reveals an unsuspected invasive adenocarcinoma in the superior segment of the right lower lobe. Note the (a,c) polylobulated solid morphology, (a,c) associated desmoplasia, and (b) internal air bronchograms.

Histopathologically, the ground-glass opacities show a lepidic growth pattern. More specifically, the cancer cells use the normal pre-existing alveolar septa as a "scaffold," growing along it without invading the stroma, pleura, or vessels. The lung cancer–screening literature also shows a higher rate of malignancy in incidental part-solid nodules compared to incidental solid nodules.

5.4 Pre-invasive Lesions

5.4.1 Atypical Adenomatous Hyperplasia

Atypical adenomatous hyperplasia (AAH) is the earliest detectable preinvasive lesion. On LDCT, AAH manifests as small ground-glass opacity, typically less than 5 mm in diameter, with no solid or part-solid component. Bronchial and vascular margins are preserved (► Fig. 5.3). Histologically, AAH is characterized by proliferation of atypical cuboidal-to-columnar epithelial cells along the alveoli and respiratory bronchioles without evidence of invasion. In the spectrum of adenocarcinoma, lesions are often multicentric. Thus, it is not uncommon for foci of AAH to be found adjacent to surgically resected invasive adenocarcinomas (IAs).

5.4.2 Adenocarcinoma In Situ

There is a continuum of morphologic change between AAH and adenocarcinoma in situ (AIS). Histologically, AIS likewise demonstrates purely lepidic growth without stromal, vascular, or pleural invasion. But on LDCT, the purely ground-glass nodular opacity of AIS is larger in size. Most AIS lesions measure between 5 and 20 mm in diameter but can be as large as 3 cm. The size of the ground-glass opacity correlates with the potential for invasion. A size threshold of less than 10 mm is often used to differentiate preinvasive lesions from potentially invasive lesions. AIS is also typically slightly greater in attenuation than AAH but still lacks solid components and manifests as pure ground glass (▶ Fig. 5.4). The differential diagnosis of subsolid nodules includes entities such as infection, focal interstitial fibrosis, and primary lung adenocarcinoma. Most ground-glass lesions resolve spontaneously. Therefore, the initial appropriate management of such lesions is simply a repeat short-term follow-up LDCT as prescribed by Lung CT Screening Reporting and Data System (Lung-RADS; Chapter 6). Persistent ground-glass opacities, however, convey a greater malignant potential than an equivalent persistent solid nodule. The differential diagnosis of persistent ground-glass opacity includes AAH, AIS, lymphoproliferative disease, focal interstitial fibrosis, and organizing pneumonia. Radiologists should pay particular attention to not only changes in size of nodular opacities on follow-up LDCT imaging, but also changes in attenuation. An increase in nodule attenuation portends an increased risk of malignancy. Multi-focal persistent ground-glass nodules are often the result of primary lung cancers or lung metastases. AAH and AIS are more frequently encountered in multiple ground-glass nodules.

5.5 Invasive Lesions

5.5.1 Minimally Invasive Adenocarcinoma

Minimally invasive adenocarcinoma (MIA) is a solitary adenocarcinoma measuring ≤ 3 cm in diameter. Unlike the preinvasive lesions, MIA does show a small invasive component of cancer cells infiltrating the myofibroblastic stroma on histopathology. Most MIAs are nonmucinous in nature. The invasive component usually measures ≤ 5 mm. MIA is excluded if there is any invasion of lymphatics, pleura, vasculature, or tumor necrosis. On LDCT, MIA appears as a part-solid nodule. The solid component may vary in size and represents the focus of invasion (▶ Fig. 5.5). Additional imaging features suggestive of invasion on LDCT include the presence of air bronchograms, spiculated or lobulated borders, pleural retraction, and/or a concave notch in the solid component. It should be stressed that mucinous and nonmucinous varieties of MIA can present as both solid and part-solid nodules on LDCT. Accurate assessment of part-solid nodules requires thin slice LDCT < 3 mm and ideally 1 to 1.5 mm. The relative size of the solid (invasive) to ground-glass (noninvasive) components ultimately determines the appropriate course of patient management and eventual prognosis. The radiologist should report the total diameter of a part-solid nodule and the diameter of its solid component. The latter should be measured on mediastinal window and level settings. Once the solid component measures 8 to 10 mm in diameter, the yield from CT-guided biopsy improves to 93%. Positron emission tomography (PET) imaging may also prove useful once the nodular component has increased to this size range.

5.5.2 Invasive Adenocarcinoma

IA demonstrates at least one focus of invasive cancer measuring greater than 5 mm in diameter. IA represents more than 70% of resected adenocarcinomas and is composed of a heterogeneous mixture of histologies (▶ Table 5.2). IA is classified according to the predominant histologic component (i.e., acinar, papillary, micropapillary, solid, lepidic). IAs are also predominantly mucinous in contrast to the predominant nonmucinous preinvasive lesions already discussed. On LDCT, IA is most often solid or predominantly solid, frequently contains internal air bronchograms, and may have a lobar or multilobar distribution (▶ Fig. 5.6).

5.6 Malignancy Rate Based on Morphology and Doubling Times

LDCT screens may reveal the presence of solid or subsolid nodules. Subsolid nodules may be purely ground glass or part solid in morphology (▶ Fig. 5.2). About 75% of solid solitary pulmonary nodules are benign. About 80% of benign solid nodules are sequelae of a granulomatous infection, 5 to 10% represent a hamartoma, and 5 to 10% of various miscellaneous etiologies. About 25% of solitary solid nodules are neoplastic, about 92% of which represent a primary lung cancer and about 8% a solitary extrathoracic metastases. Forty-two percent of these primary lung cancers are of the adenocarcinoma cell type. Twenty-two percent represent squamous cell cancers and 23% small cell or large cell lung cancers. The differential diagnosis of subsolid nodules was discussed in the previous section. In the ELCAP study, the prevalence of malignancy varied with lesion morphology on LDCT. Among the positive baseline screens, 19% of cases were a part-solid or ground-glass nodule. Among these cases, 34% of subsolid nodules were malignant as opposed to 7% of solid nodules. The rate of malignancy was highest for part-solid nodules at 63%. The malignancy rate in the pure ground-glass nodules was 18%. Even after standardizing for nodule size, the malignancy rate was statistically much higher for part-solid nodules than for either solid or ground-glass lesions (▶ Table 5.3). Most of the subsolid malignancies were adenocarcinoma spectrum lesions. However, for solid nodules, the likelihood of malignancy increases with increasing lesion diameter (▶ Table 5.4). A spiculated border or margin has a high positive predictive value of malignancy and is indicative of such in up to 90% of cases.

As LDCT screening for the early detection of lung cancer becomes more common-place, volumetric analyses, including doubling times (DT), of screen-detected lung nodules (▶ Table 5.5) and lung cancers (▶ Table 5.6) may provide more useful information to guide patient follow-up and management or intervention. DT may be divided

Table 5.3 Malignancy rate based on lesion morphology

Lesion morphology	Rate (%)
Part solid	63
Pure ground glass	18
Solid	7

Table 5.4 Nodule size and likelihood of malignancy

Nodule size (mm)	Malignancy rate (%)
>20	50
8–20	18
4–7	0.9
<3	0.2

Table 5.5 Growth rate of small lung cancers detected on low-dose computed tomography

Nodule size	Doubling time (d)
Pure ground glass	813
Part solid	457
Solid	149

Table 5.6 Doubling times based on cancer cell type

Cell type	Doubling time (d)
Small cell lung cancer	65
Non–small cell lung cancer	180
Adenocarcinoma in situ	400

into three groups: rapid (DT < 183 days), average (DT = 183–365 days), and slow (DT > 365 days). The more rapid the DT, the greater the probability of cancer and potentially more aggressive cancer. Adenocarcinoma spectrum lesions comprise about 87% of slow DT lesions. Squamous cell cancers comprise about 60% of more rapid DT lesions. By definition, nodule growth represents a change in diameter of ≥ 1.5 mm or a change in volume of at least 25%. Measuring the difference between the current measured volume and the original measured volume and dividing this difference by the original number provides the percentage of interval increase growth.

For example, if the nodule currently measures 11 mm on LDCT and it originally measured 6 mm, the percent growth between the two LDCT studies is as follows: 11 – 6 = 5 ÷ 6 = 0.83 × 100 = 83% growth between studies. Such growth implies the nodule represents a growing cancer and potentially more aggressive-behaving cancer until proven otherwise. Further investigation may necessitate PET imaging to assess the nodule's metabolic activity, biopsy, or surgical resection.

5.6.1 Intrapulmonary Lymph Nodes

Intrapulmonary lymph nodes represent about 18% of peripheral lung nodules seen on chest CT. Most intrapulmonary lymph nodes have distinct imaging features that should easily differentiate them from indeterminate or otherwise potentially more ominous lung nodules. Intrapulmonary lymph nodes typically manifest the following imaging features:
- Well circumscribed, subpleural, angular, or ovoid.
- Located below the carina.
- One to three lines radiate out from the border (dilated lymphatic channel).
- Mean diameter: 5.5 mm.

Suggested Readings

[1] Aoki T, Hanamiya M, Uramoto H, Hisaoka M, Yamashita Y, Korogi Y. Adenocarcinomas with predominant ground-glass opacity: correlation of morphology and molecular biomarkers. Radiology. 2012; 264(2):590–596

[2] Austin JH, Romney BM, Goldsmith LS. Missed bronchogenic carcinoma: radiographic findings in 27 patients with a potentially resectable lesion evident in retrospect. Radiology. 1992; 182(1):115–122

[3] Borczuk AC, Qian F, Kazeros A, et al. Invasive size is an independent predictor of survival in pulmonary adenocarcinoma. Am J Surg Pathol. 2009; 33(3):462–469

[4] Gardiner N, Jogai S, Wallis A. The revised lung adenocarcinoma classification-an imaging guide. J Thorac Dis. 2014, 6 Suppl 5:S537–S546

[5] Garfield DH, Cadranel JL, Wislez M, Franklin WA, Hirsch FR. The bronchioloalveolar carcinoma and peripheral adenocarcinoma spectrum of diseases. J Thorac Oncol. 2006; 1(4):344–359

[6] Gould MK, Fletcher J, Iannettoni MD, et al. American College of Chest Physicians. Evaluation of patients with pulmonary nodules: when is it lung cancer?: ACCP evidence-based clinical practice guidelines (2nd edition). Chest. 2007; 132(3) Suppl:108S–130S

[7] Hasegawa M, Sone S, Takashima S, et al. Growth rate of small lung cancers detected on mass CT screening. Br J Radiol. 2000; 73(876):1252–1259

[8] Henschke CI, Yankelevitz DF, Mirtcheva R, McGuinness G, McCauley D, Miettinen OS, ELCAP Group. CT screening for lung cancer: frequency and significance of part-solid and nonsolid nodules. AJR Am J Roentgenol. 2002; 178(5):1053–1057

[9] Henschke CI, Yankelevitz DF, Mirtcheva R, McGuinness G, McCauley D, Miettinen OS, ELCAP Group. CT screening for lung cancer: frequency and significance of part-solid and nonsolid nodules. AJR Am J Roentgenol. 2002; 178(5):1053–1057

[10] Kim HY, Shim YM, Lee KS, Han J, Yi CA, Kim YK. Persistent pulmonary nodular ground-glass opacity at thin-section CT: histopathologic comparisons. Radiology. 2007; 245(1):267–275

[11] Kim TJ, Goo JM, Lee KW, Park CM, Lee HJ. Clinical, pathological and thin-section CT features of persistent multiple ground-glass opacity nodules: comparison with solitary ground-glass opacity nodule. Lung Cancer. 2009; 64(2):171–178

[12] Lee HY, Goo JM, Lee HJ, et al. Usefulness of concurrent reading using thin-section and thick-section CT images in subcentimetre solitary pulmonary nodules. Clin Radiol. 2009; 64(2):127–132

[13] Lee SM, Park CM, Goo JM, et al. Transient part-solid nodules detected at screening thin-section CT for lung cancer: comparison with persistent part-solid nodules. Radiology. 2010; 255(1):242–251

[14] Lee SM, Park CM, Goo JM, Lee HJ, Wi JY, Kang CH. Invasive pulmonary adenocarcinomas versus preinvasive lesions appearing as ground-glass nodules: differentiation by using CT features. Radiology. 2013; 268(1):265–273

[15] Lee HJ, Goo JM, Lee CH, et al. Predictive CT findings of malignancy in ground-glass nodules on thin-section chest CT: the effects on radiologist performance. Eur Radiol. 2009; 19(3):552–560

[16] Li F, Sone S, Abe H, MacMahon H, Armato SG, III, Doi K. Lung cancers missed at low-dose helical CT screening in a general population: comparison of clinical, histopathologic, and imaging findings. Radiology. 2002; 225 (3):673–683

[17] Lu CH, Hsiao CH, Chang YC, et al. Percutaneous computed tomography-guided coaxial core biopsy for small pulmonary lesions with ground-glass attenuation. J Thorac Oncol. 2012; 7(1):143–150

[18] Noguchi M, Morikawa A, Kawasaki M, et al. Small adenocarcinoma of the lung. Histologic characteristics and prognosis. Cancer. 1995; 75(12):2844–2852

[19] Ost D, Fein AM, Feinsilver SH. Clinical practice. The solitary pulmonary nodule. N Engl J Med. 2003; 348(25): 2535–2542

[20] Park CM, Goo JM, Lee HJ, et al. Focal interstitial fibrosis manifesting as nodular ground-glass opacity: thin-section CT findings. Eur Radiol. 2007; 17(9):2325–2331

[21] Shah PK, Austin JH, White CS, et al. Missed non-small cell lung cancer: radiographic findings of potentially resectable lesions evident only in retrospect. Radiology. 2003; 226(1):235–241

[22] Sun S, Schiller JH, Gazdar AF. Lung cancer in never smokers–a different disease. Nat Rev Cancer. 2007; 7(10): 778–790

[23] Travis WD, Brambilla E, Noguchi M, et al. International Association for the Study of Lung Cancer/American Thoracic Society/European Respiratory Society International Multidisciplinary Classification of Lung Adenocarcinoma. J Thorac Oncol. 2011; 6(2):244–285

[24] Trigaux JP, Gevenois PA, Goncette L, Gouat F, Schumaker A, Weynants P. Bronchioloalveolar carcinoma: computed tomography findings. Eur Respir J. 1996; 9(1):11–16

[25] Wang CW, Teng YH, Huang CC, Wu YC, Chao YK, Wu CT. Intrapulmonary lymph nodes: computed tomography findings with histopathologic correlations. Clin Imaging. 2013; 37(3):487–492

[26] Wilson DO, Ryan A, Fuhrman C, et al. Doubling times and CT screen–detected lung cancers in the Pittsburgh Lung Screening Study. Am J Respir Crit Care Med. 2012; 185(1):85–89

6 Lung Cancer–Screening Results Reporting

Mark S. Parker and Leila Rezai Gharai

Summary

This chapter discusses the appropriate means of measuring both rounded and ovoid nodules detected on lung cancer–screening examinations as well as other variable morphologic descriptors. The Lung CT Screening Reporting and Data System (Lung-RADS) for the standardized reporting, description, categorization, and management of detected lesions is described. Illustrative case examples of Lung-RADS 1, 2, 3, and 4 lesions and a sample radiologic Lung-RADS report are provided.

Keywords: nodule, nodule descriptors, measurement, Lung-RADS, radiology reports

6.1 Introduction

The American College of Radiology (ACR) Lung CT Screening Reporting and Data System (Lung-RADS) has been produced by the ACR Lung Cancer Screening Committee subgroup on Lung-RADS. This data and reporting system is a quality assurance tool. It has been specifically designed to standardize the reporting, description, categorization, and management of lesions detected on screening computed tomography (CT) examinations. Lung-RADS also alleviates potential confusion in the interpretation of LDCT studies by both radiologists and clinicians and provides a means to monitor outcome among screened individuals. The first component of the Lung-RADS reporting system is a description of nodule appearance using a specific nodule lexicon and a standardized method of nodule measurement based on morphology. The second component involves the actual categorization of the detected lesion(s) on a scale of 1 to 4 based on morphologic appearance, probability of possible neoplasia, and management recommendations. The last component addresses significant incidental pulmonary or nonpulmonary findings that may impact patient care and management (Chapter 7).

6.2 Nodule Parameters and Measurement

It is not uncommon for many individuals undergoing LDCT screening to have one or more subcentimeter nodules or nodular opacities detected. We suggest that in such instances the six most ominous nodules should be formally reported by the radiologist according to the following descriptors: size, density, presence, or absence of calcium, pattern of calcification if present, presence of fat if present, shape, morphology, and location in the data set (image slice, series, and plane; ▶ Table 6.1). Although, by convention, most nodules should be described based on lung windows in the axial plane, some lesions may be better delineated or characterized on sagittal or coronal planes and can be utilized accordingly. These descriptors are extremely important in the follow-up analysis of lesions to assess stability or interval change. Although not mandated, volumetric lung nodule analysis utilizing currently available software for solid nodules is encouraged and will likely become the standard in years to come. We currently advocate volumetric lung nodule analysis for nodules ≥ 6 mm in diameter. If a given patient has additional indeterminate subcentimeter nodules on their baseline-screening exam (i.e., more than six), a generalized statement can be made in the formal

Table 6.1 Low-dose computed tomography (LDCT) lung nodule descriptor lexicon

Nodule descriptor	Morphologic parameter
Size	Average diameter
Density	Solid, part-solid, ground-glass, infectious, inflammatory
Fat	Present or absent
Shape	Ovoid or lentiform, round, triangular
Margins	Smooth, lobulated, parenchymal, juxtapleural, endobronchial
Location in data set	Image slice number, series, and plane if not axial

report as to their presence, average size or size range, and morphology. These latter nodules also need to be carefully analyzed on follow-up studies for changes in growth, number, morphology, and/or attenuation.

By convention, if the solid or ground-glass nodule is round or spherical, a routine bidirectional (point A to point B) measurement of its diameter on lung window and level settings should be reported (▶ Fig. 6.1). Alternatively, the average diameter should be reported for ovoid or lentiform nodules (▶ Fig. 6.2). As previously discussed in Chapter 5, the radiologist should record the total diameter of part-solid nodules as well

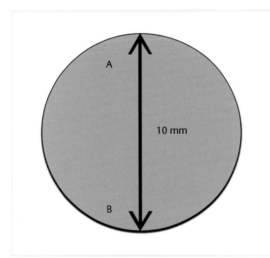

Fig. 6.1 Correct method to measure and report the dimensions of a round nodule.

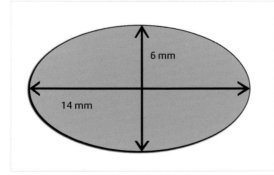

Fig. 6.2 Correct method to measure and report the dimensions of an ovoid or lentiform shaped nodule. Example: average diameter 6 + 14 = 20 ÷ 2 = 10 mm.

as the diameter of its solid component. The solid component should always be measured on mediastinal window and level settings.

6.2.1 Lung CT Screening Reporting and Data System (Lung RADS)

The ACR developed the "Lung-RADS" system for the specific reporting, follow-up, and management of both negative and positive LDCT screens. The first edition of the Lung-RADS classification scheme was modeled after the "BI-RADS" (Breast Imaging-Reporting and Data System), now in its fifth edition, long utilized for reporting screening mammography results. Like BI-RADS, Lung-RADS scores or categories are determined largely by the dominant lesion size and morphology. The size threshold for an *actionable nodule* or *positive screen* applying Lung-RADS is ≥ 6 mm for solid and part-solid nodules and ≥ 20 mm for nonsolid (ground-glass) nodules. On follow-up screening CT exams, the size cutoff is ≥ 4 mm for solid and part-solid nodules and/or an interval growth of ≥ 1.5 mm of preexisting nodule(s). New or growing nonsolid nodules must meet the ≥ 20-mm size threshold to be considered positive.

Five potential numerical Lung-RADS categories (0–4) may be assigned when reporting nodules on screening LDCT. Three modifiers ("X," "C," and "S") can also be added to any one of these numerical categories if findings other than nodules are present. The "category number" plus the "modifier code" creates the final Lung-RADS score. The "X" modifier may be used when there are additional imaging findings such as spiculated borders, a rapidly enlarging ground-glass nodule with a doubling time less than 1 year, or enlarged lymph node(s) are seen. The "S" modifier denotes the presence of additional potentially clinically significant incidental findings (e.g., coronary artery disease, emphysema, aorta aneurysm, etc.; Chapter 7). The "C" modifier applies to those screening individuals with a prior established diagnosis of lung cancer returning for follow-up for screening. It may be added to any Lung-RADS category.

Lung-RADS 0 is rarely applied in those cases in which the screening exam could not be fully completed or one in which preexisting CT studies exist but are not available to the radiologist at the time of the initial screen interpretation. This score is then modified accordingly once the study is completed or those antecedent studies become available to the radiologist for direct correlation. **Lung-RADS 1** is essentially a negative screen. That is one in which no nodules are seen on the screening exam or one that demonstrates nodules with distinctly benign patterns of calcification (e.g., completed calcified, peripheral egg shell calcifications, popcorn kernel-like central calcifications, or internal fat; ▶ Fig. 6.3). **Lung-RADS 2** is also considered a negative screen, demonstrating nodules that have a very low likelihood of becoming a clinically active cancer due to their size, morphology, or lack of growth on follow-up studies. Both **Lung-RADS 1** and **Lung-RADS 2** screen results are followed annually with repeat LDCT as long as the individual remains eligible. **Lung-RADS 3** studies are likely benign revealing nodules with a low likelihood of becoming a clinically active cancer but warrant closer surveillance with short-term follow-up imaging over 3 to 6 months for reassessment. **Lung-RADS 4** is a suspicious screen with findings representing potential lung cancer until proven otherwise. These latter cases often warrant further additional diagnostic testing (contrast-enhanced chest CT, positron emission tomography [PET]/CT) and or tissue sampling. Lung-RADS categories 0 to 4 are summarized in ▶ Table 6.2. In the vast majority of screening studies, 90% of individuals will receive a score of **Lung-RADS 1** or **2**. About 4% of individuals will receive a score of **Lung-RADS 3** and roughly 4% a

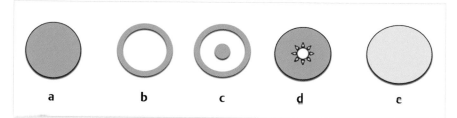

Fig. 6.3 Lung CT Screening Reporting and Data System (Lung-RADS 1) nodules: typical benign patterns of calcification or internal matrix of fat. **(a)** Completely calcified through and through-prototype: granuloma. **(b)** Peripheral rim or eggshell calcification-prototype: sarcoidosis, silicosis, partially calcified granuloma. **(c)** Target calcification-prototype: partially calcified granuloma. **(d)** Popcorn kernel or nugget of calcification-prototype: hamartoma. **(e)** Fat attenuation internal matrix-prototype: hamartoma.

Table 6.2 Simplified overview of Lung CT Screening Reporting and Data System (Lung-RADS) score and potential implications

Category	Category descriptor	Lung-RADS
Incomplete		0
Negative	No nodules or definitely benign nodules	1
Benign appearance or behavior	Nodules—very low likelihood of becoming a clinically active cancer due to size or lack of growth	2
Likely benign	Likely benign—short-term follow-up suggested; nodules—a low likelihood of becoming a clinically active cancer	3
Suspicious	Findings for which additional diagnostic testing and/or tissue sampling is recommended	4A/4B

Table 6.3 Expected distribution and probability of malignancy based on Lung CT Screening Reporting and Data System (Lung-RADS) score

Expected distribution (%)	Probability of malignancy (%)	Lung-RADS
90	< 1	1 or 2
4	1–2	3
2	5–15	4A
2	> 15	4B

Lung-RADS 4 score (▶ Table 6.3). Lung-RADS 4 is further stratified into the following: **Lung-RADS 4A**—solid nodules ≥ 8 to < 15 mm or part-solid nodules ≥ 8 mm with solid component ≥ 6 and < 8 mm; **Lung-RADS 4B**—solid nodules ≥ 15 mm or part-solid nodules with solid component ≥ 8 mm; and **Lung-RADS 4X**, which basically represents either category 3 or 4 nodules with additional features suspicious of malignancy (e.g., lymphadenopathy). The nodule with the highest individual Lung-RADS score ultimately defines the final assigned Lung-RADS category. "S" and "C" modifiers may also be applied to any Lung-RADS score on initial baseline and follow-up screens. A comprehensive breakdown of the Lung-RADS categories, description, imaging findings, management recommendations, probability of malignancy, and estimated prevalence in the screening population is provided in ▶ Table 6.4, and is also directly available

Table 6.4 Comprehensive Lung CT Screening Reporting and Data System (Lung-RADS™ Version 1.0 assessment categories release date: April 28, 2014)

Category	Category descriptor	Category	Findings	Management	Probability of malignancy	Estimated population prevalence
Incomplete	–	0	Prior chest CT(s) being located for comparison. Part or all of lungs cannot be evaluated	Additional lung cancer screening CT images and/or comparison to prior chest CT exams needed	N/A	1%
Negative	No nodules or definitely benign nodules	1	• No lung nodules • Nodule(s) with specific patterns of calcifications (e.g., complete, central, popcorn, concentric rings) and fat-containing nodules	Continue with annual LDCT screening in 12 mo	<1% (combined categories 1 and 2)	90% (combined categories 1 and 2)
Benign appearance or behavior	Nodules with a very low likelihood of becoming a clinically active cancer due to size or lack of growth	2	• Solid nodule(s): <6-mm diameter on baseline imaging or <4-mm diameter on follow-up imaging • Part-solid nodule(s): <6-mm total diameter on baseline imaging • Nonsolid nodule(s) GGN: <20 or ≥20 mm and stable or slowly growing • Category 3 or 4 nodules stable ≥3 mo	Continue with annual LDCT screening in 12 mo		
Probably benign	Probably benign lesion—short-term follow-up suggested; includes nodules with a low likelihood of becoming a clinically active cancer	3	• Solid nodule(s): ≥6 or <8-mm diameter at baseline imaging or new 4- or <6-mm diameter on follow-up imaging • Part-solid nodule(s): ≥6-mm total diameter with solid component; <6 mm on baseline imaging or new <6-mm total diameter nodule on follow-up imaging • Nonsolid nodule(s) GGN: ≥20-mm diameter in baseline imaging • Category 3 or 4 nodules stable ≥3 mo	Follow-up LDCT in 6 mo	1–2%	5%

Table 6.4 continued

Category	Category descriptor	Category	Findings	Management	Probability of malignancy	Estimated population prevalence
Suspicious	Findings that may warrant additional diagnostic testing and/or tissue sampling	4A	• Solid nodule(s); ≥ 8 or < 15 mm on baseline imaging or growing < 8 mm or new 6 or < 8 mm • Part solid nodule(s); ≥ 6 mm total diameter with solid component ≥ 6 or < 8 mm on baseline imaging or with a new or growing nodule < 4- mm solid component • Endobronchial nodule	3-mo follow-up LDCT PET/CT may be used when there is a ≥ 8-mm solid component	5–15%	2%
		4B	• Solid nodule(s); ≥ 15-mm diameter or new or growing and ≥ 8 mm • Part-solid nodule(s): Solid component ≥ 8 mm or a new or growing ≥ 4-mm solid component	• Chest CT with or without contrast • PET/CT and/or tissue sampling depending on probability of malignancy and comorbidities • PET/CT may be used when there is a ≥ 8-mm solid component	> 15%	2%
		4X	Category 3 or 4 nodules with additional findings or imaging features increasing suspicion for malignancy			
Other	Clinically significant or potentially clinically significant findings (non–lung cancer)	S	Modifier—may add on to category 0–4 codes	As appropriate to the specific finding	N/A	10%

47

Table 6.4 continued

Category	Category descriptor	Category	Findings	Management	Probability of malignancy	Estimated population prevalence
Prior lung cancer	Modifier for patients with a prior diagnosis of lung cancer who return to screening	C	Modifier—may add on to category 0–4 codes	–	–	–

Abbreviations: CT, computed tomography; GGN, ground-glass nodule; LDCT, low-dose computed tomography; PET, positron emission tomography.

Source: Modified with Permission of ACR.

Notes: (1) Negative screen: does not mean that an individual does not have lung cancer. (2) Size: nodules should be measured on lung windows and reported as the average diameter rounded to the nearest whole number; for round nodules, only a single diameter measurement is necessary. (3) Size thresholds: apply to nodules at first detection, and that grow and reach a higher size category. (4) Growth: an increase in size of > 1.5 mm. (5) Exam category: each exam should be coded 0–4 based on the nodule(s) with the highest degree of suspicion. (6) Exam modifiers: S and C modifiers may be added to the 0–4 categories. (7) Lung cancer diagnosis: once a patient is diagnosed with lung cancer, further management (including additional imaging such as PET/CT) may be performed for purposes of lung cancer staging; this is no longer screening. (8) Practice audit definitions: a negative screen is defined as categories 1 and 2; a positive screen is defined as categories 3 and 4. (9) Category 4B management: this is predicated on the probability of malignancy based on patient evaluation, patient preference, and risk of malignancy; radiologists are encouraged to use the McWilliams et al assessment tool when making recommendations. (10) Category 4X: nodules with additional imaging findings that increase the suspicion of lung cancer, such as spiculation, GGN that doubles in size in 1 year, enlarged lymph nodes, etc. (11) Nodules with features of an intrapulmonary lymph node should be managed by mean diameter and the 0–4 numerical category classification. (12) Category 3 and 4A nodules that are unchanged on interval CT should be coded as category 2, and individuals returned to screening in 12 months.

through the ACR at their Web site (https://www.acr.org/~/media/ACR/Documents/PDF/QualitySafety/Resources/LungRADS/AssessmentCategories.pdf).

6.3 Illustrative Lung Cancer Screen Report

A sample of a standard lung cancer–screening CT report that we use is provided in ▶ Fig. 6.4. Notice the differences between this report and that of a standard chest CT report. The report should be identified as either an **initial** or a **baseline screen** versus an **annual follow-up screen**. We then break our lung cancer–screening report down into six broad categories. The first category, **Clinical Indications**, stipulates that the individual meet the current eligibility criteria for screening. Although not mandatory, our program coordinator collects additional demographic information during her initial lung assessment screening interview, which we include in this section such as age when the individual began smoking, whether or not one or both parents smoked, positive family history of lung cancer, and exposure to various potential lung carcinogens (e.g., hard metals, radon asbestos, etc.). The second category records the **CTDI$_{vol}$** (CT dose index) and **DLP** (dose length product) of the exam. We also record the individual's height, weight, and BMI (body mass index) in this section. This information is useful in monitoring radiation dose. The third section is a succinct **Summation Statement** regarding the **Lung Cancer Screening Results** (Lung-RADS score or category), recommended next step in management based on the Lung-RADS score, and the identification of potentially clinically significant findings detected on the screen (Chapter 7). At this early step in the report, we have provided all the necessary information the referring physician and screenee need regarding the screening results and what to do next. The remaining sections provide a more detailed description of the imaging findings. In particular, the fourth section is a detailed description of the **Lung Cancer-Screening**

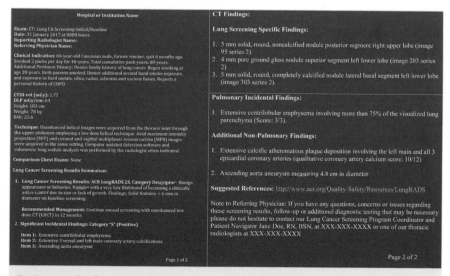

Fig. 6.4 Sample of a standard 2-page lung cancer screening computed tomography report currently used at the authors' institution.

Findings utilizing the nodule lexicon described earlier in this chapter and addressing specific nodule location based on lobe, segment, slice image, and series number. The latter is obviously important in documenting stability or changes on follow-up screens performed. The fifth section describes **Incidental Pulmonary Findings** such as the presence and degree of centrilobular or other forms of emphysema, small airways disease, bronchiectasis, etc. (Chapter 7). The sixth section describes **Additional Incidental Nonpulmonary Findings** that may be of clinical importance (e.g., presence, degree, and extent of coronary artery calcifications, adrenal or thyroid lesions, aneurysms, etc.; Chapter 7). We complete the report with a link to the ACR Lung-RADS Web site should the referring physician require more information regarding the screen category and management as well as direct contact information to our lung cancer–screening program coordinator and patient navigator to address any additional questions or management issues.

6.4 Illustrative Lung-RADS Examples

This next section will go through a series of early detection lung cancer–screening exams and a description of the pertinent imaging findings to highlight the Lung-RADS system and its appropriate application:

- Lung-RADS 1 nodules: ▶ Fig. 6.5; ▶ Fig. 6.6.
- Lung-RADS 2 nodules: ▶ Fig. 6.7, ▶ Fig. 6.8, ▶ Fig. 6.9.
- Lung-RADS 3 nodules: ▶ Fig. 6.10, ▶ Fig. 6.11, ▶ Fig. 6.12.
- Lung-RADS 4 nodules: ▶ Fig. 6.13, ▶ Fig. 6.14, ▶ Fig. 6.15, ▶ Fig. 6.16, ▶ Fig. 6.17, ▶ Fig. 6.18.
- "S" modifier (also see Chapter 7): ▶ Fig. 6.19.

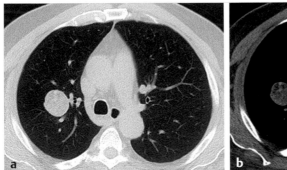
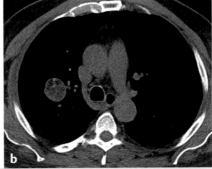

Fig. 6.5 (a) Axial low-dose computed tomography (LDCT lung windows) from the baseline screening exam of a 67-year-old man show a well-defined rounded solid nodule in the right upper lobe. On the **(b)** accompanying soft-tissue windows, the nodule contains fat consistent with a benign hamartoma. The benign features of this nodule categorize it a Lung CT Screening Reporting and Data System (Lung-RADS) category 1 lesion. The recommended management is annual screening with LDCT.

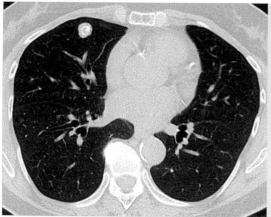

Fig. 6.6 Axial low-dose computed tomography (LDCT) image from the baseline screen of a 71-year-old woman shows a solid nodule in the right middle lobe. This nodule demonstrates popcorn calcification, consistent with a benign hamartoma. The benign features of this nodule categorize it a Lung CT Screening Reporting and Data System (Lung-RADS) category 1 lesion. The recommended management is annual screening with LDCT.

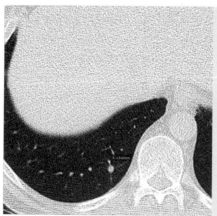

Fig. 6.7 Axial low-dose computed tomography (LDCT) image of a 63-year-old man shows a 5-mm solid rounded nodule in the posterior basal segment right lower lobe. Solid nodules < 6 mm in diameter on baseline LDCT are classified as Lung CT Screening Reporting and Data System (Lung-RADS) category 2 nodules, that is, nodules with a benign appearance or behavior. The recommended management is annual screening with LDCT.

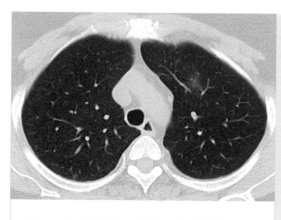

Fig. 6.8 Axial low-dose computed tomography (LDCT) of a 56-year-old woman shows a 16-mm nonsolid (ground-glass) nodule in the anterior segment left upper lobe on baseline screening. Nonsolid nodules measuring < 20 mm in diameter on baseline LDCT are classified as Lung CT Screening Reporting and Data System (Lung-RADS) category 2 nodules. That is, nodules with a benign appearance or behavior. The recommended management is annual screening with LDCT.

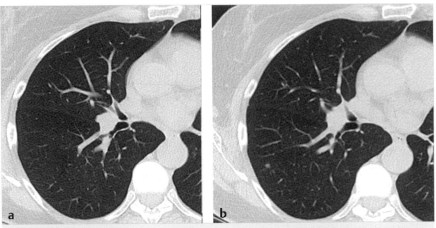

a b

Fig. 6.9 (a) Baseline and (b) annual follow-up low-dose computed tomography (LDCT) screen of a 62-year-old woman. (a) Baseline screen was negative. (b) Annual follow-up screen shows a new 3-mm solid nodule in the right lower lobe. New solid nodules measuring < 4 mm in diameter on annual screening exams have a very low likelihood of becoming malignant and are classified as Lung CT Screening Reporting and Data System (Lung-RADS) category 2 nodules. The recommended management is annual screening with LDCT.

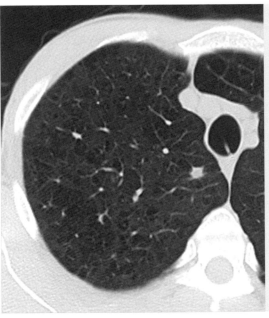

Fig. 6.10 Axial low-dose computed tomography (LDCT) screen of a 58-year-old man shows a 6-mm solid nodule in the medial aspect posterior segment right upper lobe on baseline screening. Solid nodules measuring ≥ 6 mm in diameter on baseline LDCT are classified as Lung CT Screening Reporting and Data System (Lung-RADS) category 3, probably benign nodules but warrant more close surveillance. Follow-up LDCT in 6 months is recommended to document stability. Note the extensive centrilobular emphysema.

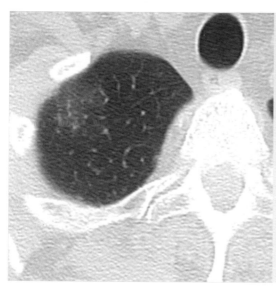

Fig. 6.11 Axial low-dose computed tomography (LDCT) screen of a 63-year-old man shows a 22-mm nonsolid (ground-glass) nodule in the right upper lobe on baseline screening. Nonsolid nodules measuring ≥ 20 mm on baseline LDCT are classified as Lung CT Screening Reporting and Data System (Lung-RADS) category 3, probably benign. Follow-up LDCT in 6 months is recommended to document stability.

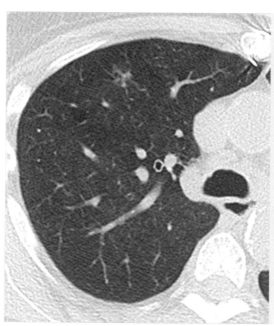

Fig. 6.12 Axial low-dose computed tomography (LDCT) screen of a 74-year-old woman shows an 8-mm part-solid nodule with a 3-mm solid component (mediastinal window measurement, not illustrated) in the right upper lobe on baseline screening. Part-solid nodules measuring ≥ 6 mm total diameter with solid component < 6 mm are classified as Lung CT Screening Reporting and Data System (Lung-RADS) category 3, probably benign. Reassessment on LDCT in 6 months is recommended for reassessment.

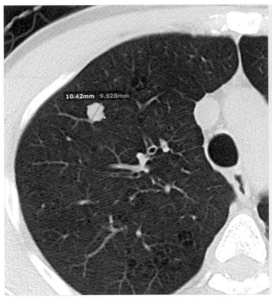

Fig. 6.13 Axial low-dose computed tomography (LDCT) screen of a 58-year-old man shows a 10-mm solid, round, slightly lobulated noncalcified nodule in the right upper lobe on baseline screening. Solid nodules measuring ≥ 8 mm but < 15 mm are classified as Lung CT Screening Reporting and Data System (Lung-RADS) category 4A (suspicious for neoplasia). Further evaluation with additional diagnostic testing such as PET (positron emission tomography)/CT or tissue sampling is advised in such cases.

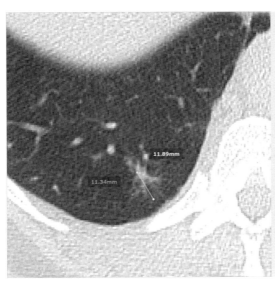

Fig. 6.14 Axial low-dose computed tomography (LDCT) screen of a 71-year-old woman shows a 12-mm part-solid nodule with a 6-mm solid component (mediastinal window measurement, not illustrated) in the posterior basal segment right lower lobe on baseline screening. Part-solid nodules measuring ≥ 6 mm total diameter with solid component ≥ 6 to < 8 mm are classified as Lung CT Screening Reporting and Data System (Lung-RADS) category 4A (suspicious for neoplasia). Further evaluation with additional imaging such as PET (positron emission tomography)/CT or tissue sampling is advised in such cases.

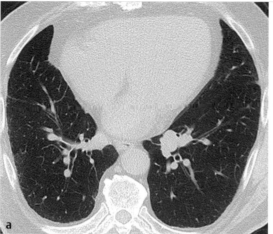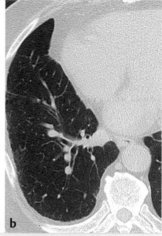

a   b

Fig. 6.15 (a,b) Axial LDCT screen of a 75-year-old man shows a rounded noncalcified endobronchial nodule in the mid posterior basal bronchus of the right lower lobe on baseline screening. Endobronchial nodules are classified as Lung CT Screening Reporting and Data System (Lung-RADS) category 4A (suspicious for neoplasia). Further evaluation with additional diagnostic imaging exams such as PET (positron emission tomography)/CT, octreotide scan, and/or tissue sampling is advised in such cases.

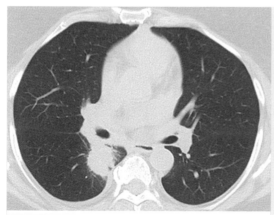

Fig. 6.16 Axial low-dose computed tomography (LDCT) screen of a 72-year-old woman shows a 28-mm solid noncalcified lobulated nodule in the medial superior segment right lower lobe on baseline screening. Solid nodules measuring ≥ 15 mm are classified as Lung CT Screening Reporting and Data System (Lung-RADS) category 4B (suspicious nodules). Further evaluation with additional diagnostic testing such as PET (positron emission tomography)/CT or tissue sampling is advised in such cases.

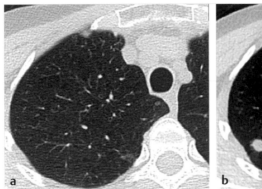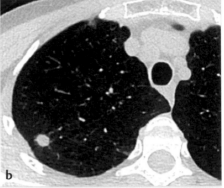

a b

Fig. 6.17 Axial low-dose computed tomography (LDCT) screen of a 66-year-old man. The baseline screening was Lung CT Screening Reporting and Data System (Lung-RADS) category 2 because of a 10-mm pure ground-glass nodule in the medial posterior segment of the **(a)** right upper lobe. **(b)** A new 8-mm solid nodule in the posterior segment right upper lobe on annual follow-up screening. A new nodule ≥ 8 mm on subsequent screening is considered suspicious for neoplasia. The examination is reclassified as a Lung-RADS category 4B. Further evaluation with PET (positron emission tomography)/CT scan or tissue sampling is recommended.

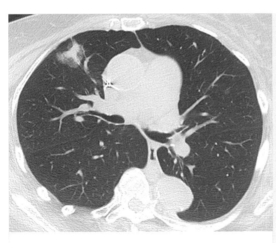

Fig. 6.18 Axial low-dose computed tomography (LDCT) screen of a 79-year-old woman shows a lobulated 27-mm part-solid nodule with a solid component measuring 15 mm (mediastinal window measurement, not illustrated) in the right upper lobe on baseline screening. Note the associated spiculated margins and pleural tails, which make this nodule highly suspicious (a Lung CT Screening Reporting and Data System [Lung-RADS] category 4X nodule). Further evaluation with additional diagnostic imaging such as PET (positron emission tomography)/CT and/or tissue sampling is recommended.

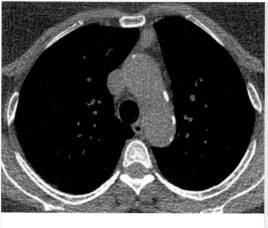

Fig. 6.19 Axial low-dose computed tomography (LDCT) screen (mediastinal windows) of a 69-year-old woman shows an incidental solid nodule in anterior mediastinum. Category S modifier is added on to category 0–4 Lung CT Screening Reporting and Data System (Lung-RADS) scores when appropriate. The suggested management includes clinical correlation and further evaluation with cross-sectional imaging and or tissue sampling. This is in addition to the appropriate management for the specified Lung-RADS category. Diagnosis: incidental thymoma.

Suggested Readings

[1] Moyer VA, U.S. Preventive Services Task Force. Screening for lung cancer: U.S. Preventive Services Task Force recommendation statement. Ann Intern Med. 2014; 160(5):330–338

[2] Aberle DR, Adams AM, Berg CD, et al. National Lung Screening Trial Research Team. Reduced lung-cancer mortality with low-dose computed tomographic screening. N Engl J Med. 2011; 365(5):395–409

[3] American College of Radiology. Lung CT Screening Reporting and Data System (Lung-RADS). Available at: http://www.acr.org/Quality Safety/Resources/LungRADS

[4] Fintelmann FJ, Bernheim A, Digumarthy SR, et al. The 10 pillars of lung cancer screening: rationale and logistics of a lung cancer screening program. Radiographics. 2015; 35(7):1893–1908

[5] Gierada DS, Pinsky P, Nath H, Chiles C, Duan F, Aberle DR. Projected outcomes using different nodule sizes to define a positive CT lung cancer screening examination. J Natl Cancer Inst. 2014; 106(11):106

[6] Henschke CI, Yip R, Yankelevitz DF, Smith JP, International Early Lung Cancer Action Program Investigators*. Definition of a positive test result in computed tomography screening for lung cancer: a cohort study. Ann Intern Med. 2013; 158(4):246–252

[7] American College of Radiology. Lung CT Screening Reporting and Data System (Lung-RADS™). Available at: https://www.acr.org/quality-safety/resources/lungrads

[8] MacMahon H, Austin JH, Gamsu G, et al. Fleischner Society. Guidelines for management of small pulmonary nodules detected on CT scans: a statement from the Fleischner Society. Radiology. 2005; 237(2):395–400

[9] National Comprehensive Cancer Network. NCCN Clinical Practice Guidelines in Oncology. 2016 Lung Cancer Screening Version 1. Fort Washington, PA: National Comprehensive Cancer Network; 2017. Available at: https://www.nccn.org/professionals/physician_gls/pdf/lung_screening.pdf

[10] Naidich DP, Bankier AA, MacMahon H, et al. Recommendations for the management of subsolid pulmonary nodules detected at CT: a statement from the Fleischner Society. Radiology. 2013; 266(1):304–317

[11] Aberle DR, Adams AM, Berg CD, et al. National Lung Screening Trial Research Team. Reduced lung-cancer mortality with low-dose computed tomographic screening. N Engl J Med. 2011; 365(5):395–409

[12] Manos D, Seely JM, Taylor J, Borgaonkar J, Roberts HC, Mayo JR. The Lung Reporting and Data System (LU-RADS): a proposal for computed tomography screening. Can Assoc Radiol J. 2014; 65(2):121–134

7 Detection and Management of Unexpected Incidental Pulmonary and Nonpulmonary Findings

Robert C. Groves, Mark S. Parker, and Avinash Pillutla

Summary

This chapter focuses on some of the more commonly encountered incidental pulmonary and nonpulmonary findings encountered on lung cancer screens, highlighting typical CT (computed tomography) imaging findings as well as the potential clinical implications of such. The qualitative visual or ordinal scoring of the extent of centrilobular emphysema, coronary artery calcifications, and osteoporosis with compression fractures are discussed in detail with illustrative case examples.

Keywords: incidental finding, unexpected finding, COPD, coronary artery disease, osteoporosis, pulmonary Langerhans' cell histiocytosis, respiratory bronchiolitis, desquamative interstitial pneumonia, acute eosinophilic pneumonia, thyroid, ordinal score, Agatston

7.1 Introduction

As any radiologist can attest, incidental findings are quite prevalent on radiologic exams and can often distract from the original clinical intent, leaving both the radiologist and referring clinician unsure of the next appropriate step in management. Whereas most screening tests only include information about one particular organ system (e.g., mammography: breast; prostate-specific antigen [PSA]: prostate; colonoscopy: colon), lung cancer screening (LCS) with low-dose computed tomography (LDCT) provides a great deal of information about other organ systems outside the realm of possible lung cancer. Erb et al reported the rate of non-nodule incidental findings was as high as 67% in their series. The detection of incidental findings, however, should not necessarily be regarded as a downside of LCS CT. Besides assessing for the presence or absence of lung nodules, LDCT screening is an opportunity to screen for other conditions that can adversely impact a given individual's health including but not limited to chronic obstructive pulmonary disease (COPD), coronary artery disease, and osteoporosis. This may in fact further increase its cost-effectiveness and provide better global outcomes. The interpreting radiologist and referring physician must be prepared to recognize, address, and know how to handle the additional "incidental" information afforded by LCS. To further complicate matters, LCS also often reveals challenging lung abnormalities specific to the current and former smoking population that can mimic more ominous diseases, including potential lung cancer. The characterization of other nonpulmonary lesions (e.g., thyroid, adrenal, etc.) may also prove difficult on LDCT due to quantum mottle, excessive noise, and lack of intravenous iodinated contrast media. This chapter will focus on some of the more commonly encountered incidental pulmonary and nonpulmonary findings encountered on lung cancer screens, highlighting typical CT imaging findings as well as potential clinical implications.

7.2 Incidental Pulmonary Findings: Smoking-Related Lung Diseases

7.2.1 Chronic Obstructive Lung Disease

COPD, including chronic bronchitis and emphysema, is a major cause of morbidity and mortality in LCS populations and the fourth leading cause of death. Twenty percent of smokers develop COPD, so it is vital we identify those screened individuals at increased risk of such and quantify or at least qualify the extent of emphysema. The low-dose technique of LCS CT is designed to depict high-attenuation structures such as lung nodules, not low-attenuation process such as emphysematous lung. Additionally, the iterative reconstruction algorithms employed to reduce radiation dose may also "hamper" the depiction of emphysematous lung. Therefore, accurate quantification of emphysema may be somewhat limited on these studies. However, qualitative assessment, especially of moderate and extensive emphysema is possible and may be used as a potential risk stratification tool. At our institution, we visually score the extent of centrilobular emphysema and rate it on a scale of 0 to 3: 0 (none)—no centrilobular emphysema appreciated; 1 (mild)—centrilobular emphysema involving less than 25% of the visualized lung parenchyma; 2 (moderate)—centrilobular emphysema involving greater than 25% but less than 50% of the visualized lung parenchyma; and 3 (severe)—centrilobular emphysema involving greater than 50% of the visualized lung parenchyma. Although not mandated, we chose to report emphysema scores greater than 1 as significant findings ("S" modifier) in addition to our Lung CT Screening Reporting and Data System (Lung-RADS) score (► Table 7.1). Other institutions may opt to report the degree of emphysema in other manners. Some representative case examples applying this qualitative emphysema scoring system are illustrated in ► Fig. 7.1, ► Fig. 7.2, ► Fig. 7.3.

In addition to emphysema, several additional lung parenchymal abnormalities directly result from tobacco abuse. Examples include pulmonary Langerhans' cell histiocytosis (PLCH) and the spectrum of interstitial pneumonias ranging from respiratory bronchiolitis-interstitial lung disease (RB-ILD) to desquamative interstitial pneumonia (DIP). Acute eosinophilic pneumonia (AEP) has also been linked to cigarette smoking in some studies, although smoking is likely only one of numerous causes and not a definitive causative agent alone. The basis for all smoking-related lung diseases is predominately an inflammatory response. The inflammation is caused by the numerous noxious antigens found in cigarette smoke followed by the body's attempt at repairing the resultant damage. Cigarette smoke produces a powerful inflammatory response stimulating an increased influx of macrophages and other anti-inflammatory cells into the lungs. This ultimately results in destruction of lung tissue, followed by attempted reparation through the deposition of collagen and fibrous tissue. The latter is directly

Table 7.1 Qualitative emphysema score on lung cancer screens ("S" modifier)

Extent of emphysema	Score
No visualized emphysema	0
Emphysema involving < 25% of the visualized lung parenchyma	1
Emphysema involving > 25%, but < 50% of the visualized lung parenchyma	2
Emphysema involving > 50% of the visualized lung parenchyma	3

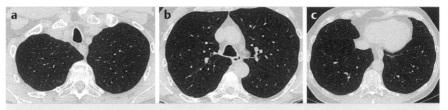

Fig. 7.1 Selected low-dose computed tomography (LDCT) screen images through the **(a)** upper, **(b)** mid-, and **(c)** lower lung zones reveal a mild degree of centrilobular emphysema involving less than 25% of the visualized lung parenchyma. Qualitative score: 1/3. Note the saber sheath trachea **(a)**.

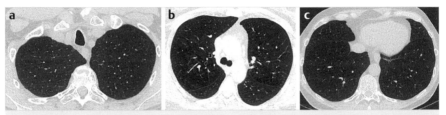

Fig. 7.2 Selected low-dose computed tomography (LDCT) screen images through the **(a)** upper, **(b)** mid-, and **(c)** lower lung zones reveal a moderate degree of centrilobular emphysema involving more than 25% but less than 50% of the visualized lung parenchyma. Qualitative score: 2/3.

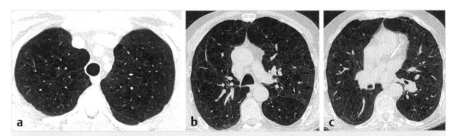

Fig. 7.3 Selected low-dose computed tomography (LDCT) screen images through the **(a)** upper, **(b)** mid-, and **(c)** lower lung zones reveal an extensive degree of centrilobular emphysema involving more than 50% of the visualized lung parenchyma. Qualitative score: 3/3.

proportional to the amount of cigarette smoking incurred by the individual. Eventually, with continued smoking, irreversible fibrosis occurs in the alveolar walls, causing the syndrome now known as combined pulmonary fibrosis and emphysema. The latter is often complicated by pulmonary hypertension. These smoking-related lung diseases have typical CT imaging features the radiologist can apply to establish the appropriate diagnosis. Many of the histopathologic and imaging findings associated with these various smoking-related diseases improve with smoking cessation and abstinence.

7.2.2 Pulmonary Langerhans' Cell Histiocytosis

PLCH is a rare smoking-related disorder typically seen in young adults in the third to fourth decade of life. Symptomatic patients may present with dyspnea, nonproductive cough, and fatigue. Secondary spontaneous pneumothorax occurs in about 15% of individuals. A small percentage of individuals are entirely asymptomatic and diagnosed solely because of incidentally detected imaging findings. Histologically, PLCH is characterized by granulomatous infiltration of the distal bronchioles. Although the diagnosis may be suggested with high accuracy on CT, the evolving nature and wide variety of imaging findings associated with PLCH can sometimes prove challenging. When imaging is inconclusive, tissue biopsy may be necessary for a definitive diagnosis.

As with most smoking-related lung disorders, the mid and upper lung zones are predominately affected in PLCH. Early in the disease process, the most common imaging manifestation is ill-defined micronodularity in a peribronchial and centrilobular distribution. Typically, the nodules measure less than 1.0 cm in size and some may have subtle surrounding ground glass or central cavitation. As active inflammation decreases, the nodular pattern dissipates and is replaced by more thick-walled cysts. These cysts gradually lose wall thickness, increase in size, coalesce, and become more bizarre and irregular in shape and morphology as the disease progresses. End-stage fibrosis is a rare long-term complication. Remember PLCH is an evolving disease and as such a constellation of these imaging findings may coexist in any given patient. When CT reveals both nodules and bizarre shaped cysts in a young smoker, the diagnosis is highly suggested. In the early nodular phase, PLCH may be indistinguishable from RB or endobronchial spread of infection. In the cystic phase, the differential diagnosis might include *Pneumocystis* pneumonia or LAM (lymphangioleiomyomatosis), depending on the clinical scenario. Serial imaging exams and appropriate history are invaluable in establishing the correct diagnosis. More than 50% of PLCH patients experience complete spontaneous resolution or stabilization without treatment; even better results are reported with smoking cessation. The latter is the recommended first line of management for PLCH. Corticosteroids may be of some benefit in the early stages of the disease. In a minority of cases, the disease progresses to end-stage fibrosis, at which time lung transplantation may be the only viable option.

7.2.3 Respiratory Bronchiolitis (Also Known as "Smoker's Bronchiolitis")

RB is histopathologically characterized by an accumulation of pigmented macrophages and inflammation without fibrosis involving the respiratory bronchioles. It affects nearly all cigarette smokers. Interestingly, RB is typically asymptomatic and only discovered incidentally on imaging, if at all. Rarely, heavier smokers, with more than 30 pack-years of abuse, may develop symptomatic RB-ILD. Individuals with RB-ILD are usually young and complain of chronic cough and progressive dyspnea over 1 to 2 years. Bibasilar, end-inspiratory crackles or crackles throughout inspiration and sometimes into early expiration may be auscultated. RB-ILD is occasionally diagnosed in former smokers and in persons exposed to secondhand smoke or fumes. Pulmonary function tests (PFTs) may be normal but alternatively may reveal an increased residual volume, mixed obstructive-restrictive pattern, mild hypoxemia, and mild to moderate reduction in the diffusion capacity for carbon monoxide (DLCO). On CT, the imaging findings of RB and RB-ILD are inseparable. In most instances, CT will be normal. In

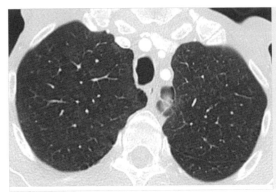

Fig. 7.4 Select low-dose computed tomography (LDCT) screen axial image through the upper lung zones of a current asymptomatic heavy cigarette smoker reveals diffuse albeit subtle ill-defined centrilobular ground-glass nodules heavily concentrated in the upper lobes. Note the saber sheath trachea reflecting underlying COPD (chronic obstructive pulmonary disease). Diagnosis: respiratory bronchiolitis.

others, CT may demonstrate poorly defined centrilobular nodules (71%) and ground-glass opacities (67%; ► Fig. 7.4). Although more profuse in the upper lung zones (53%), the mid and lower lung zones may be affected (20%). Bronchial wall thickening is seen in nearly all persons with RB-ILD (90%). Most persons also have concomitant mild centrilobular emphysema (57%). Air trapping is not uncommon on expiratory images. Fibrotic changes manifest by intralobular linear opacities and honeycombing is only seen in about 25% of persons diagnosed with RB-ILD. RB-ILD may coexist with clinical and imaging findings of DIP, another smoking-related disease, discussed later in this chapter. Other potential diseases that may have a similar CT imaging appearance include subacute hypersensitivity pneumonitis, nonspecific interstitial pneumonitis (NSIP), and early PLCH. First-line treatment of RB-ILD entails smoking cessation, which typically results in either improvement or stabilization of the symptoms. RB-ILD does not typically progress to end-stage pulmonary fibrosis in most persons.

7.2.4 Desquamative Interstitial Pneumonia

Among the smoking-related interstitial lung diseases, DIP represents the end of the RB-ILD spectrum. Histopathologically, DIP is characterized by diffuse, marked intra-alveolar accumulation of macrophages and minimal interstitial fibrosis. Like RB-ILD, DIP is uncommon and typically affects younger to middle-aged adult cigarette smokers. Unlike RB-ILD, DIP is seen nearly twice as often in males. Although approximately 90% of persons diagnosed with DIP are current or former cigarette smokers, a similar histopathologic pattern has been described in various metabolic diseases, drug reactions, connective tissue disorders, and cases of dust inhalation. Most affected persons present with acute pulmonary symptoms, and have more mild pulmonary function abnormalities than those diagnosed with usual interstitial pneumonia (UIP). Affected persons complain of cough and dyspnea. PFTs often reveal a restrictive pattern and hypoxemia. On CT, the predominant imaging finding is peripheral, lower lung zone ground-glass opacities (► Fig. 7.5). However, DIP may also manifest as widespread or patchy distributed foci of ground glass as well. Small cystic spaces can be seen within the foci of ground glass, reflecting early fibrosis (► Fig. 7.6). Honeycombing is not a typical feature. The imaging features of DIP are often nonspecific and may overlap with the appearance of other entities, including RB-ILD, NSIP, and organizing pneumonia (OP). Therefore, in the appropriate clinical setting, biopsy may be warranted to confirm the diagnosis. Ultimately, patients with DIP have a good prognosis with cessation of smoking and

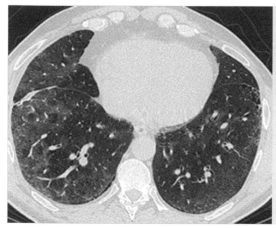

Fig. 7.5 Select low-dose computed tomography (LDCT) screen axial image through the lower lung zones of a current asymptomatic heavy cigarette smoker reveals predominantly basilar juxtapleural ground-glass opacities. Diagnosis on open lung biopsy: desquamative interstitial pneumonia.

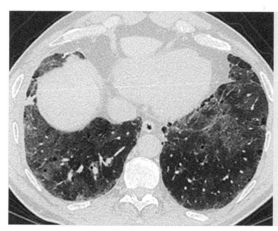

Fig. 7.6 Select low-dose computed tomography (LDCT) screen axial image through the lower lung zones of a current asymptomatic heavy cigarette smoker reveals predominantly basilar juxtapleural ground-glass opacities and scattered subcentimeter cystic lesions reflective of early fibrosis. Diagnosis on open lung biopsy: desquamative interstitial pneumonia.

corticosteroid therapy. With continued smoking, however, progressive disease and even death have been documented.

7.3 Incidental Nonpulmonary Findings

7.3.1 Coronary Artery Calcifications

Current and former smokers are at increased risk of both lung cancer and coronary heart disease (CHD). Coronary artery calcification (CAC) increases with both tobacco use and increasing age. The presence of any CAC increases mortality. About 25% of National Lung Screening Trial (NLST) participants succumbed to CHD. Semi-automated Agatston CAC scoring on cardiac-gated CT allows early risk stratification of those persons at increased risk. The ungated low-dose LCS technique, however, obviates accurate Agatston CAC scoring. However, numerous studies have shown analogous benefits from a visual qualitative analysis of CAC extent to identify high-risk persons. The use of an ordinal visual score on LCS CT has also been shown to correlate well with the four major

Table 7.2 Qualitative CAC (coronary artery calcification) score on lung cancer screens ("S" modifier)

Visualized extent of epicardial CAC	Score
No visualized calcification	0
Calcification involving less than one-third the length of the entire artery	1
Calcification involving more than one-third but less than two-thirds the length of the entire artery	2
Calcification involving more than two-thirds the length of the entire artery	3
Total qualitative CAC score	X/12

Agatston score categories routinely used on dedicated calcium scoring CT. Given the significant prognostic implications of the presence or absence of CAC, performing a visual qualitative calcium score on all LCS CTs is encouraged and has been shown to have high concordance between radiologists.

Visual qualification of CAC assesses the four major epicardial coronary arteries: left main, left anterior descending, circumflex, and right coronary artery. The qualitative score for each of the four epicardial coronary arteries can be divided into four categories: none (0)—no visualized epicardial CAC; mild (1)—calcification involving less than one-third the length of the entire artery; moderate (2)—calcification involving more than one-third but less than two-thirds the length of the artery; and severe (3)—calcification involving more than two-thirds the length of the artery. A total qualitative ordinal score for all four vessels (0–12) can then be reported (▶ Table 7.2; ▶ Fig. 7.7). Using CAC score of 0 as a reference, a total CAC score of at least 4 has been shown to be a significant predictor of potential cardiovascular death (odds ratio 4.7). Those screened persons with moderate or severe CAC scores (≥4) may benefit from a formal medical assessment for complete risk stratification and management that could potentially decrease their risk of a significant adverse cardiovascular event. At our institution, we

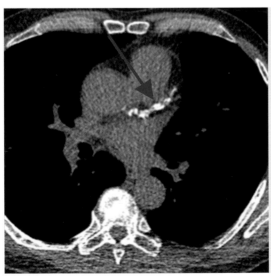

Fig. 7.7 Select low-dose computed tomography (LDCT) screen axial image through the mediastinum of a current asymptomatic heavy cigarette smoker reveals extensive calcification in the left main and left anterior descending coronary artery territories. Both vessels receive a qualitative score of 3/3. This may portend a potential increased risk of an adverse cardiovascular event in this person. The circumflex and right coronary arteries demonstrated moderate CAC (coronary artery calcification) as well (not illustrated).

routinely report the presence or absence of CAC and include total qualitative scores ≥ 4 as a significant finding ("S" modifier) in addition to our Lung-RADS score. Other institutions may opt to report the degree of CAC in other manners.

7.3.2 Thyroid Lesions

Chest CT identifies more incidental thyroid nodules (ITNs) than any other imaging modality. Unfortunately, there is no definitive reliable CT imaging feature to distinguish between benign and malignant nodules. As such, these incidentally detected thyroid nodules are a frequent diagnostic conundrum for both radiologists and referring clinicians. Incidentally detected thyroid nodules present even more of a diagnostic challenge on LCS CT due to increased quantum mottle accentuated by the low-dose technique. Inappropriate workup of these thyroid nodules may lead to increased anxiety for screened individuals as well as costly unnecessary diagnostic tests and potential biopsies. While some potential for malignancy exists in these frequently encountered thyroid nodules, most are actually benign. Of those thyroid nodules that prove to be malignant, most of these tend to have an indolent course. Fortunately, many publications have emerged on the management of incidental detected thyroid nodules and a consensus on whether or not to pursue further diagnostic evaluation has been reached. This consensus is based on both the imaging appearance of the thyroid nodule and specific patient demographics. Nodule size is the CT imaging feature primarily used to direct potential further management. Current guidelines suggest further evaluation with ultrasound should be pursed for ITN > 1.0 cm in axial dimension if the individual is less than 35 years of age and for ITN > 1.5 cm if the individual is 35 years or older (i.e., the latter reflecting the LCS population; ▶ Fig. 7.8). These criteria assume that no additional suspicious imaging features are present (e.g., regional lymphadenopathy, local invasion by the nodule). If additional suspicious imaging findings are present, ultrasound evaluation is warranted regardless of nodule size or the individual's age. Furthermore, no additional diagnostic workup of an ITN is recommended when no suspicious findings are present or in those persons with significant comorbidities, unless that person has known risk factors for thyroid cancer or otherwise specifically requested by the referring clinician.

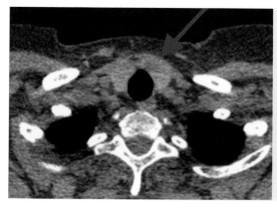

Fig. 7.8 Select low-dose computed tomography (LDCT) screen axial image through the thoracic inlet and upper mediastinum of an asymptomatic former heavy cigarette smoker reveals an ill-defined 1.5-cm low-attenuation lesion in the left thyroid lobe. Further evaluation with ultrasonography (not illustrated) and subsequent biopsy revealed papillary carcinoma.

7.3.3 Osteoporosis

Current and former heavy cigarette smokers have an increased risk of lung, head and neck, bladder, and other cancers, COPD, CHD, and osteoporosis. These diseases may all coexist in this population and may share a common pathophysiology. Although vertebral fractures are prevalent in more than 10% of the general adult population, the prevalence of vertebral body fractures and decreased vertebral body attenuation or bone density on sagittal reconstructed LDCT lung cancer screens are independently associated with all-cause mortality. Buckens et al reported the prevalence of vertebral fractures at 35 to 51% in their screening population. They further reported that the prevalence of vertebral body fractures and lower bone density on screening populations was associated with a doubling of the risk (adjusted hazard ratio [HR]: 2.04 [1.43–2.92]) for all-cause mortality independent of age, smoking status, pack-years smoked, coronary and aortic calcification, and volume and severity of emphysema. Vertebral body fractures are readily visible on sagittal LCS LDCT reconstructions and can be scored with good reliability. Utilizing Genant's semiquantitative vertebral fracture assessment method, Buckens et al described vertebral body fractures according to the percentage of vertebral body height loss at that level compared to an adjacent normal vertebra. The investigators graded compression fracture severity as follows: grade 1—mild loss of height (20–25%); grade 2—moderate loss of height (25–40%); and grade 3—severe loss of height (> 40%; ▶ Table 7.3). Buckens et al further stratified their data by analyzing the worst fracture grade and a cumulative fracture category. The worst fracture grade was defined as the worst fracture visible (maximum grade 3). The cumulative fracture score was the sum of all recorded fracture scores. The latter were then categorized into one of three categories: 0—no fractures; 1 to 3—mild cumulative fracture burden; or ≥ 4—moderate to severe cumulative fracture burden (▶ Fig. 7.9). Recent publications have also shown that CT attenuation values in the trabecular region of vertebral bone correlate with dual-energy X-ray absorptiometry (DXA) values. Again, this serves as a potential viable marker for osteoporosis and potential bisphosphonate therapy aiming to reduce fracture risk and to reduce all-cause mortality. For each 10 HU (Hounsfield units) decline in trabecular bone attenuation, the adjusted HR is about 1.08 (1.02–1.15). CT attenuation values are best measured on axial images in trabecular regions of the vertebral bodies away from the cortex at either L1 or the nearest visible, unfractured, relatively normal-appearing vertebral body. The region of interest should avoid bone islands, traversing vessels, and hemangiomas. Obviously lower HU reflect less dense and higher risk bone and thus greater mortality.

Table 7.3 Vertebral body compression score on sagittal lung cancer screens ("S" modifier)

Vertebral body compression score	Score
Height preserved or < 20% loss of height	0
Mild: 20–25% loss of height	1
Moderate: 25–40% loss of height	2
Severe: > 40% loss of height	3

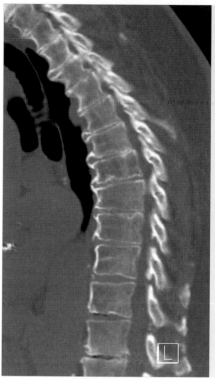

Fig. 7.9 Select low-dose computed tomography (LDCT) screen sagittal multiplanar reconstruction (MPR; bone window) image through the thoracic spine an asymptomatic current heavy cigarette smoker reveals mild compression deformities of T7 and T8 with 20 to 25% loss of vertebral body height. The total cumulative fracture burden is likewise mild.

Suggested Readings

[1] American Thoracic Society, European Respiratory Society. American Thoracic Society/European Respiratory Society International Multidisciplinary Consensus Classification of the Idiopathic Interstitial Pneumonias. This joint statement of the American Thoracic Society (ATS), and the European Respiratory Society (ERS) was adopted by the ATS board of directors, June 2001 and by the ERS Executive Committee, June 2001. Am J Respir Crit Care Med. 2002; 165(2):277–304

[2] Attili AK, Kazerooni EA, Gross BH, Flaherty KR, Myers JL, Martinez FJ. Smoking-related interstitial lung disease: radiologic-clinical-pathologic correlation. Radiographics. 2008; 28(5):1383–1396, discussion 1396–1398

[3] Bartalena T, Giannelli G, Rinaldi MF, et al. Prevalence of thoracolumbar vertebral fractures on multidetector CT: underreporting by radiologists. Eur J Radiol. 2009; 69(3):555–559

[4] Bolland MJ, Grey AB, Gamble GD, Reid IR. Effect of osteoporosis treatment on mortality: a meta-analysis. J Clin Endocrinol Metab. 2010; 95(3):1174–1181

[5] Brauner MW, Grenier P, Tijani K, Battesti JP, Valeyre D. Pulmonary Langerhans cell histiocytosis: evolution of lesions on CT scans. Radiology. 1997; 204(2):497–502

[6] Buckens CF, van der Graaf Y, Verkooijen HM, et al. Osteoporosis markers on low-dose lung cancer screening chest computed tomography scans predict all-cause mortality. Eur Radiol. 2015; 25(1):132–139

[7] Buckens CF, de Jong PA, Mol C, et al. Intra and interobserver reliability and agreement of semiquantitative vertebral fracture assessment on chest computed tomography. Woloschak GE, ed. PLoS ONE. 2013; 8:e71204

[8] Castoldi MC, Verrioli A, De Juli E, Vanzulli A. Pulmonary Langerhans cell histiocytosis: the many faces of presentation at initial CT scan. Insights Imaging. 2014; 5(4):483–492

[9] https://www.cdc.gov/copd/maps/docs/pdf/MD_COPDFactSheet.pdf. Accessed August 2, 2017

[10] Centers for Disease Control and Prevention (CDC). Annual smoking-attributable mortality, years of potential life lost, and productivity losses—United States, 1997–2001. MMWR Morb Mortal Wkly Rep. 2005; 54(25): 625–628

[11] Chan PL, Reddy T, Milne D, Bolland MJ. Incidental vertebral fractures on computed tomography. N Z Med J. 2012; 125(1350):45–50

[12] Erb CT, Sather P, Michaud GC, Detterbeck FC, Tanoue LT. Incidental Findings Discovered in a Lung Cancer Screening Program. B61: Managing Lung Cancer Screening and its Downstream Findings. Thematic Poster Session, American Thoracic Society International Conference, May, 2017

[13] Galvin JR, Franks TJ. Smoking-related lung disease. J Thorac Imaging. 2009; 24(4):274–284

[14] Genant HK, Wu CY, van Kuijk C, Nevitt MC. Vertebral fracture assessment using a semiquantitative technique. J Bone Miner Res. 1993; 8(9):1137–1148

[15] Hoang JK, Langer JE, Middleton WD, et al. Managing incidental thyroid nodules detected on imaging: white paper of the ACR Incidental Thyroid Findings Committee. J Am Coll Radiol. 2015; 12(2):143–150

[16] Hogg JC, Chu F, Utokaparch S, et al. The nature of small-airway obstruction in chronic obstructive pulmonary disease. N Engl J Med. 2004; 350(26):2645–2653

[17] Marshall HM, Bowman RV, Yang IA, Fong KM, Berg CD. Screening for lung cancer with low-dose computed tomography: a review of current status. J Thorac Dis. 2013; 5 Suppl 5:S524–S539

[18] Mets OM, de Jong PA, Prokop M. Computed tomographic screening for lung cancer: an opportunity to evaluate other diseases. JAMA. 2012; 308(14):1433–1434

[19] Müller D, Bauer JS, Zeile M, Rummeny EJ, Link TM. Significance of sagittal reformations in routine thoracic and abdominal multislice CT studies for detecting osteoporotic fractures and other spine abnormalities. Eur Radiol. 2008; 18(8):1696–1702

[20] Mueller-Mang C, Grosse C, Schmid K, Stiebellehner L, Bankier AA. What every radiologist should know about idiopathic interstitial pneumonias. Radiographics. 2007; 27(3):595–615

[21] Park JS, Brown KK, Tuder RM, Hale VA, King TE, Jr, Lynch DA. Respiratory bronchiolitis-associated interstitial lung disease: radiologic features with clinical and pathologic correlation. J Comput Assist Tomogr. 2002; 26 (1):13–20

[22] Parker MS, de Christenson RL, Abbott GF. Diffuse lung disease: desquamative interstitial pneumonia (DIP). In: Chest Imaging Case Atlas. 2nd ed. New York, NY: Thieme; 2012:531–533

[23] Parker MS, de Christenson RL, Abbott GF. Diffuse lung disease: respiratory bronchiolitis-interstitial lung disease. In: Chest Imaging Case Atlas. 2nd ed. New York, NY: Thieme; 2012:568–570

[24] Parker MS, de Christenson RL, Abbott GF. Diffuse lung disease: pulmonary Langerhans cell histiocytosis. In: Chest Imaging Case Atlas. 2nd ed. New York, NY: Thieme; 2012:578–581

[25] Patel AR, Wedzicha JA, Hurst JR. Reduced lung-cancer mortality with CT screening. N Engl J Med. 2011; 365 (21):2035–, author reply 2037–2038

[26] Pickhardt PJ, Pooler BD, Lauder T, del Rio AM, Bruce RJ, Binkley N. Opportunistic screening for osteoporosis using abdominal computed tomography scans obtained for other indications. Ann Intern Med. 2013; 158(8): 588–595

[27] Romme EA, Murchison JT, Phang KF, et al. Bone attenuation on routine chest CT correlates with bone mineral density on DXA in patients with COPD. J Bone Miner Res. 2012; 27(11):2338–2343

[28] Shemesh J, Henschke CI, Shaham D, et al. Ordinal scoring of coronary artery calcifications on low-dose CT scans of the chest is predictive of death from cardiovascular disease. Radiology. 2010; 257(2):541–548

[29] Watanabe K, Fujimura M, Kasahara K, et al. Acute eosinophilic pneumonia following cigarette smoking: a case report including cigarette-smoking challenge test. Intern Med. 2002; 41(11):1016–1020

[30] Watanabe R, Tatsumi K, Hashimoto S, Tamakoshi A, Kuriyama T, Respiratory Failure Research Group of Japan. Clinico-epidemiological features of pulmonary histiocytosis X. Intern Med. 2001; 40(10):998–1003

[31] Watts JR, Jr, Sonavane SK, Snell-Bergeon J, Nath H. Visual scoring of coronary artery calcification in lung cancer screening computed tomography: association with all-cause and cardiovascular mortality risk. Coron Artery Dis. 2015; 26(2):157–162

[32] Williams AL, Al-Busaidi A, Sparrow PJ, Adams JE, Whitehouse RW. Under-reporting of osteoporotic vertebral fractures on computed tomography. Eur J Radiol. 2009; 69(1):179–183

[33] Woo EK, Mansoubi H, Alyas F. Incidental vertebral fractures on multidetector CT images of the chest: prevalence and recognition. Clin Radiol. 2008; 63(2):160–164

8 Elements of a Successful Lung Cancer–Screening Program

Mark S. Parker, Joanna E. Kusmirek, and Michelle Futrell

Summary

This chapter succinctly describes those key elements that must be implemented for lung cancer–screening programs of any size and volume to be successful and impact the care of potential screenees. Key components including but not limited to eligibility criteria, education of screenees, providers, radiologists, appropriate computed tomography (CT) image acquisition and interpretation, radiation dose, reporting, and communication of pertinent findings are discussed. The currently approved billing codes for reimbursement purposes are also provided. This chapter also provides an in-depth discussion on smoking cessation counseling techniques including behavioral modification, motivational interviewing, change talk, nicotine replacement therapy with patches, lozenges, and nasal sprays as well as currently approved medications that may be used to help smokers quit smoking.

Keywords: best practice parameters, eligibility, multidisciplinary team, navigator-coordinator, self-referral, reimbursement, shared decision making, CTDIvol, DLP, American Association of Physicists in Medicine, computer-assisted detection, volumetric nodule analysis, Dutch–Belgian Randomized Lung Cancer Screening Trial, CMS registry, quality control, smoking cessation counseling, ACR designation, Patient Protection and Affordable Care Act, CPT codes, G-codes, ICD-10 diagnosis codes, nicotine replacement therapy, bupropion, varenicline

8.1 Introduction

In order to be truly successful and positively impact the lives of millions of high-risk persons, today's lung cancer–screening (LCS) programs must provide a level of care and continuity in care similar to that of the original 33 medical centers participating in the National Lung Screening Trial (NLST). Best practice parameters have been developed by the American College of Radiology (ACR) in collaboration with the Society of Thoracic Radiology (STR) to assist medical facilities in meeting these goals and expectations. Radiologists actively involved or participating in LCS programs are encouraged to read, follow, and apply these best practice parameters. Similarly, the American College of Chest Physicians (ACCP) and the American Thoracic Society (ATS) released policy statements addressing the same that are also available for review. Additionally, Fintelmann et al published a key article in 2015 in which the authors discussed what they referred to as the "10 pillars of successful LCS." Programs or practices involved in LCS for the early detection of lung cancer are also encouraged to read and apply the concepts outlined in the Fintelmann et al article.

8.2 Key Components to Making Your LCS Program Work

The following section addresses some key components we found important at our institution for the initial establishment, subsequent growth, and eventual success of our early detection LCS program. Programs contemplating the development or further growth of an LCS program need to realize the importance of not only reaching out to their neighboring community of potential eligible screenees, but also establishing a firm cohesive relationship with their primary health care providers and referrals. It is also important to have a close working relationship with a multidisciplinary team of specialists and subspecialists, either within your own institution or in close proximity to it, highly invested in the early detection, management, and treatment of not only early-stage lung cancer, but also other "lung health" issues. LCS programs also require the full support from radiology administrators, chairpersons, and the hospital administration in order to succeed. We will now briefly address some key components that were helpful in our LCS program and hopefully will likewise be helpful in setting up your own program.

8.2.1 Screenee Eligibility

Screening only those eligible at-risk persons is paramount. The current eligibility requirements for LCS mandated for reimbursement purposes by the Centers for Medicare & Medicaid Services (CMS) were briefly addressed in Chapter 4. Once again, CMS approves low-dose computed tomography (LDCT) LCS for asymptomatic Medicare beneficiaries aged 55 to 77 years with a history of heavy tobacco abuse. Heavy tobacco abuse is defined as current smokers with a 30-pack-year history of abuse or the equivalent thereof or former smokers with an equivalent smoking history having quit within the past 15 years. CMS does restrict the age of eligible Medicare persons to 55 to 77 years as opposed to 80 years recommended by the U.S. Preventive Services Task Forces (USPSTF). Most private third-party payers now follow either the CMS or USPSTF eligibility requirements for reimbursement. It should be noted that other medical societies have proposed similar but different LCS eligibility criteria. For example, the ACCP, American Society of Clinical Oncology (ASCO), ATS, American Cancer Society (ACS), and the American Lung Association (ALA) all endorse screening for asymptomatic former and current smokers aged 55 to 74 years, similar to the original NLST participants. Although National Comprehensive Cancer Network (NCCN) stratifies their eligibility requirements to asymptomatic smokers 55 to 74 years with the same pack-year history of abuse, it also considers younger current or formers smokers ≥ 50-years of age, with less of a tobacco abuse history, namely 20 pack-years, who also have additional risk factors, such a personal history of emphysema or pulmonary fibrosis, personal history of various cancers or occupational exposure to known carcinogens (e.g., asbestos, radon), or a family history of lung cancer (NCCN 2 criteria). Our institution currently follows both the USPSTF and CMS eligibility guidelines but also considers the latter NCCN 2 criteria in certain circumstances. However, programs should realize that at this time, NCCN 2 eligibility criteria are not typically reimbursable.

8.2.2 Screenee, Provider, and Radiologist Education

Appropriate education regarding the rationale and logistics of LCS is a key element to the success of any LCS program. Education involves not only the individual undergoing screening, but also the radiologists, primary care providers, and hospital administrators and leadership. The shared decision making (SMD) process (Chapter 4) is specifically designed and developed to educate the individual contemplating screening. The shared decision making process should be supplemented by written or virtual visual aids or pamphlets that contain similar information to that presented in the SMD described in layman terms. Radiologists must be well trained in the acquisition and interpretation of high-quality low-dose chest exams, the use and application of the nodule lexicon or nomenclature, and reporting screen results by application of the Lung CT Screening Reporting and Data System (Lung-RADS). Primary care-providers may receive educa tion about LCS through one-on-one conversations, group meetings, conferences, grand rounds, newsletters, and online materials. Every LCS program should maintain an updated Web page that includes frequently asked questions (FAQs) for prospective individuals contemplating screening and providers as well as direct links to educational material provided by the ACR (https://www.acr.org/Quality-Safety/Resources/Lung-Imaging-Resources), Lung Cancer Alliance (ww.lungcanceralliance.org/am-i-at-risk/), NCCN (https://www.nccn.org/patients/guidelines/lung_screening/), and/or the ACS (https://www.cancer.org/latest-news/who-should-be-screened-for-lung-cancer.html). It is also helpful to differentiate those persons who may be eligible for LCS but may not be candidates for such using a potential risk calculator. A direct link to http://www.shoul-discreen.com is a very helpful resource for both primary care providers and individuals to assist them in this personal process. It is also essential that hospital administrators and leaders ensure the allocation of space and time, and clerical, nursing, physician staffing as well as financial resources needed to sustain and grow the LCS program. Even low-volume LCS programs will need the monetary funds to hire and train qualified support staff, purchase state-of-the-art equipment, information technology, and patient tracking software. With increasing screening volume and follow-up screens and studies, the need for additional CT technologists and CT scanners, radiologists (possibly with thoracic imaging training or interventional skills), pulmonologists, and thoracic surgeons must also be both anticipated and supported.

LCS is not something to be taken lightly. It is not an exam or procedure. LCS is a "process" that involves a "team." It is imperative that all members of this multidisciplinary team, including the individual being screened, understand that this is not a "one time and your done screen" but rather a "long-term process." In particular, it is a "process" that most likely will go on for decades for most screened individuals, their primary care providers, the radiologists, and the screening center. The LCS multidisciplinary team must be well educated in lung health and the many nuances of lung disease, including diseases that may mimic lung cancer, and in the diagnosis and management of screen-detected lung cancer. Central to every LCS program team are the coordinator and navigator(s) who interact with each and every facet of the program (▶ Fig. 8.1). This includes interfacing with the referring primary care services, securing preauthorization for reimbursement purposes, CT schedulers, insurers, CMS, determining screening eligibility or pursuing a diagnostic exam in appropriate cases, relaying and following up on screen results to the referral service and/or screened individual, orchestrating appropriate annual or shorter term interval follow-up exams and/or intervention if needed, offering and/or ensuring smoking cessation counseling is provided, and uploading data into the mandatory CMS registry. The LCS program coordinator and navigators may be a midlevel provider (e.g., physician assistant [PA] or nurse practitioner [NP]) working under the supervision of a physician in the department of radiology, medicine, or surgery. An LCS program cannot and will not succeed without heavily invested and competent program coordinators and patient navigators.

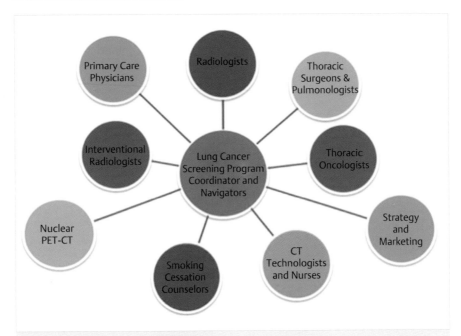

Fig. 8.1 Spoke wheel diagram illustrating some of the key stakeholders in a successful lung cancer–screening program. Central to every program, regardless of its size, are the Program Coordinator and Navigators(s) who interact with every other stakeholder invested in the program as well as the screened individual to ensure optimal results and outcome.

8.2.3 LDCT Screening Ordering Process and Self-Referrals

Only a physician or a qualified nonphysician practitioner (e.g., PA, NP, or clinical nurse specialist [CNS]) can submit an order for LDCT LCS as mandated by CMS. The order and screening exam can only be performed "after" provided documentation that the individual meets the eligibility requirements and that both parties participated in the shared decision making process. Radiology departments can ensure compliance of this process by integrating this documentation process into the interface of their specific computerized order entry systems. It should be acknowledged that both the ACR and STR practice parameters provide provisions allowing medical centers to accept self-referrals for LCS with LDCT at the discretion of the facility director. However, facilities accepting self-referrals are required to have mechanisms in place to refer these particular persons to qualified health care providers to address and manage abnormal screen results. Additionally, self-referrals are not reimbursable by CMS.

8.3 Acquiring the LDCT Screen Images

The ACR-STR has developed basic imaging requirements and parameters for LCS with LCDT that imaging centers and radiologists must follow. These practice parameters include the following:
- Minimum 16-detector CT scanner.
- Unenhanced helical technique performed at full inspiration.

- Z-axis should cover the lung apices through the costophrenic angles.
- Slice thickness ≤ 2.5 mm (1 mm preferred).
- Gantry rotation ≥ 500 ms per rotation.
- Radiation dose should be "as low as reasonably achievable" without compromising diagnostic quality. Maximum threshold dose **CTDI$_{vol}$**: 3 mGy for a standard-sized patient (5.7 feet [170 cm]; weight, 155 lb [69.75 kg]) employing "appropriate dose reduction" for smaller persons and "appropriate dose increases" for larger persons. For a typical scan length of 35 cm, the dose length product or **DLP** (CTDI$_{vol:}$ × scan length) is about 105 mGy/cm (note: at our institution, we routinely report the screened individual's height, weight, BMI [body mass index], and the CTDI$_{vol}$ and DLP in the report; ▶ Fig. 6.4).
- Maximum intensity projection (MIP) images may be used to facilitate nodule detection.
- The American Association of Physicists in Medicine provides sample low-dose imaging protocols for most major CT vendors that may be accessed online at http://www.aapm.org/pubs/CTProtocols/documents/LungCancerScreeningCT.pdf.

8.3.1 LDCT Screen Image Interpretation

CMS stipulates that only those physicians with documented training in diagnostic radiology and radiation safety can interpret LDCT LCS examinations and claim reimbursement for such. The interpreting physician must be either board certified or board eligible by the American Board of Radiology (ABR) or an equivalent organization. Additional criteria the interpreting physician must satisfy include their participation in continuing medical education (CME) in accordance with ACR standards and personal involvement in the supervision or interpretation of at least 300 chest CTs in the preceding 3 years. All acquired LCS CT images should be reviewed and interpreted on an acceptable picture archiving and communication system (PACS) workstation. MIP as well as multiplanar reconstruction (MPR) images can be used to facilitate nodule detection. Approved computer-assisted detection (CAD) software can be employed as needed as a second but not as a primary reader. The standard is to report lung nodules detected on contiguous axial images (lung windows) using the previously described nodule lexicon (▶ Table 6.1) and measuring techniques described earlier (▶ Fig. 6.1; ▶ Fig. 6.2). However, detected lesions may be reported on any imaging plane that best depicts the dimensions and morphologic features of the nodule of concern. If volumetric software is available, such can be used to assess the percentage of nodule growth (or decrease) and potentially nodule doubling times where appropriate. As previously discussed in Chapter 6 and as reported in the Dutch–Belgian Randomized Lung Cancer Screening Trial (NELSON), a volume increase of at least 25% after at least 3 months is a reliable indicator of interval growth. On both interim and annual follow-up screens, the radiologist should always analyze all previously described or reported antecedent nodules for interval changes in size, shape, attenuation, or dimensions as well as report the presence of new nodules or unexpected incidental findings that might otherwise impact the individual care and management (Chapter 7).

8.3.2 Concise Communication of the LDCT Screen Findings

The clear, concise reporting of the observed imaging findings on the initial baseline, interim, and annual follow-up LDCT screens is of paramount importance to guide referral services in the appropriate management of their patient and to minimize unnecessary diagnostics workups, procedures, and the overall incurred radiation dose. The radiologist should always report the LCS imaging findings in accordance with the Lung-RADS system (Chapter 6) using a standardized template or format (e.g., ▶ Fig. 6.4). It is also helpful to include in the report a direct link to the ACR Lung-RADS reporting system (https://www.acr.org/~/media/ACR/Documents/PDF/QualitySafety/Resources/LungRADS/AssessmentCategories.pdf) to ensure the referral service and screened individual clearly understand the screen results and how those results should be appropriately managed. Despite all of the imaging findings that may be observed by the radiologist, screened individuals and the referral services basically want the answers to three questions: (1) Is there or is there not cancer present? (2) Is there anything else bad going on in the chest that I need to know about? (3) What do I need to do next? The radiologist needs to be certain his or her report clearly answers these three questions or concerns. At our institution, individuals may enroll in the LCS program via a dedicated outpatient LCS clinic. A face-to-face discussion occurs with the screened individual following the radiologist's review of the exam and discussion of the findings with a pulmonologist staffing the clinic. In some cases, both the radiologist and pulmonologist review the imaging findings together with the screened individual. The referral service receives a hard copy of the final report and a CD (compact disc) of the screen if the latter is desired. Some category 3 cases and all category 4 results are discussed directly with the referring physician over the telephone. Our institution also allows patients to directly access their final reports via an electronic patient portal within 2 days if they so wish.

8.4 Multidisciplinary Team

As stressed earlier, a successful LCS program does not involve only a few persons, but rather an entire network or multidisciplinary team of lung specialists fully invested in the early diagnosis and management of patients not only with possible lung cancer, but also with all forms of lung disease (▶ Fig. 8.1). If such a team of specialists does not exist at the screening center, it is critical that screened persons and the referring physicians have access to a nearby network of clinicians that can provide such support. It is also critical that smoking cessation is part of this multidisciplinary approach. Once an individual has actually committed to come in and enroll in an LCS program, they may be more willing than ever before to seriously consider cessation counseling. LCS provides a unique "teachable moment" for individuals undergoing screening, especially if they have the opportunity to see their screening images firsthand and witness the deleterious effects smoking may be having on their lungs and coronary arteries. Smoking cessation can substantially reduce the risk of lung cancer and at the same time increase the cost-effectiveness of screening by 20 to 45%. Local smoking cessation resources can also be used in LCS programs to further supplement material available online through the Centers for Disease Control and Prevention, ACS, ALA, and NCCN.

8.5 Centers for Medicare & Medicaid Services Registry and Quality Control

The ACR developed a CMS-approved National Lung Cancer Screening Registry in May 2015. Data can be submitted into the registry retroactively on lung cancer screens performed on or after January 1, 2015. It should be stressed that CMS requires monitoring of *all* screened persons, both those with Medicare and those with private insurance, to be downloaded into this registry. One of the many roles of this registry is recording data on smoking history, radiation dose, downstream care, interventions performed, and complications related to such, for both local and national auditing and benchmarking. Centers performing LCS examinations should also consider becoming accredited by the ACR as a Designated Lung Cancer Screening Center. The ACR Lung Cancer Screening Center designation is a further testament to the neighboring community, prospective patients, patients, and referral services that the LCS program and team have an unwavering commitment to providing the highest level of medical and radiologic expertise in the screening, early detection, and management of lung cancer.

8.6 Reimbursement for LDCT Screens

As a result of the grade B recommendation by the USPSTF, under section 2713 of the Patient Protection and Affordable Care Act, all third-party insurers are required by law to cover the cost of LCS LDCT for those persons meeting the eligibility requirements, without co-pay, deductible, or coinsurance. CMS reimbursement for LCS, and by default that for many third-party payers, is currently directly related to the following five issues:
- Are only eligible persons being screened?
- Is the screen performed and interpreted correctly?
- Are the findings and recommendations being appropriately conveyed to the referring primary health care provider?
- Is there a mechanism in place by which screened individuals receive appropriate follow-up and management?
- Are specific data points being collected, tracked, and downloaded into the CMS registry?

Currently, there are two "**G-codes**" used for the screening process:
- **G0296**: Counseling and shared decision-making visit to discuss the need for LCS.
- **G0297**: LDCT scan for LCS itself.

The **S8032** code that was previously used by private payers is now obsolete. At the time of this writing, all payers should use the **G0297** code for the LDCT scan for LCS.
The **ICD-10** diagnosis codes are somewhat more complicated. CMS currently limits the allowable **ICD-10** diagnosis codes that can accompany claims for both **G0296** and **G0297** to the following:
- **Z87.891** (personal history of nicotine dependence).
- **F17.210** (nicotine dependence, cigarettes, uncomplicated).
- **F17.211** (nicotine dependence, cigarettes, in remission).
- **F17.213** (nicotine dependence, cigarettes, with withdrawal).
- **F17.218** (nicotine dependence, cigarettes, with other nicotine-induced disorders).
- **F17.219** (nicotine dependence, cigarettes, with other unspecified nicotine-induced disorders).

It is important to realize that the above **Z code** for *former smokers* and *cigarette-specific* **F-codes** for *current smokers* are the **only** **ICD-10** codes that CMS will currently accept for **G0296** and **G0297** claims at the time of this writing. If **any** other diagnosis code is added to a CMS claim, even when the above allowable codes are also used, some LCS program claims may be rejected.

Some private payers may require the use of **ICD-10** code **Z12.2** (encounter for screening for malignant neoplasm for respiratory organs) for LCS claims. Also, some private payers will accept other **F-codes** that are not specific to cigarettes, such as **F17.20** (nicotine dependence, unspecified) or **F17.290** (nicotine dependence, other tobacco product, uncomplicated), which CMS will not accept.

In summary, coders currently have two basic options depending upon the payer. CMS limits the diagnosis codes to only Z87.891, F17.210, F17.211, F17.213, F17.218, or F17.219, and when it is a private payer, use whatever array of **ICD-10** codes that will appropriately meet the payer's standard of medical necessity.

There has also been a change in the smoking and tobacco use cessation codes. Until recently, there were two separate sets of tobacco cessation counseling visit codes: **CPT 99406** and **CPT 99407** for symptomatic patients, and **G0436** and **G0437** for asymptomatic patients. However, as of October 1, 2016, there is no longer a distinction between symptomatic and asymptomatic individuals. The two **G-codes** for cessation counseling have been eliminated, and **CPT 99406** and **CPT 99407** should be used for cessation counseling regardless of whether the patient has signs or symptoms of tobacco-related disease (personal communication, Lung Cancer Alliance, December 19, 2016).

8.7 Expansion of At-Risk Populations for LDCT Screens

Compared with other screening exams that have been in use for many years, LCS with LDCT is in its infancy. Undoubtedly, as more national demographic and benchmark data are collected, eligibility criteria beyond smoking history and age alone using other forms of risk stratification and perhaps even serum biomarkers will play more of an integral role (Chapter 9). These factors along with further identification of nodule morphologic features associated with higher rates of malignancy may impact screening intervals, screening duration, and result in even earlier detection of occult lung cancers and further improve outcomes.

8.8 Smoking Cessation Counseling

CMS requires that health care providers stress the importance of cigarette smoking abstinence for former smokers and of smoking cessation for current smokers and to also provide tobacco cessation interventions. As discussed in Chapter 2, cigarette smoking is the number one risk factor for lung cancer and the leading cause of preventable death in the United States. The benefits of quitting are numerous and the effect on the body is almost instantaneous; within 20 minutes of smoking the last cigarette, the heart rate and blood pressure begin to decrease. Just 1 year after quitting, the risk of coronary artery disease is half that of a smoker. Five years after quitting, the risk of several cancers is reduced by half, or is normal risk, and after 10 to 15 years the likelihood of dying of lung cancer is cut in half.

Smoking cessation must involve a two-pronged, comprehensive approach to quitting: one addresses the pharmacological aspect of smoking and the other the behavioral aspect of smoking. Evidence shows that smokers are more successful at quitting when nicotine replacement therapy (NRT) is provided in conjunction with behavioral counseling. NRT helps reduce one's dependence on nicotine, by titrating the patient from a higher dose of nicotine to a lower dose over time. Behavioral counseling is designed to identify and disassociate behavioral triggers that form the habit of smoking and focus on one's motivations for quitting.

Proven successful in eliciting change in behavior, motivational interviewing (MI) is a behavioral counseling technique with practical application to smoking cessation counseling. *MI* is a counseling style centered on the individual. Its aim is to help the individual resolve ambivalence about behavior change. The approach is not one of coercion to change, but rather a conversation that is rooted in respect, compassion, and acceptance to help uncover their motivation or desire to quit smoking and evoke positive statements or change talk. *Change talk* is any expression from the individual that favors change. The goal is to have the individual recognize a discrepancy exists between their current behavior and their personal goals and values. For example, during a conversation they might express they think being a smoker is not a good example for their children. The discrepancy that exists is their desire to be a good role model for their children and their current smoking habit. The discrepancy is likely to increase the level of motivation they feel toward quitting.

OARS is an acronym that stands for **Open-Ended Questions, Affirmations, Reflections,** and **Summaries**. *OARS* is an important communication skill used in engaging and throughout MI. These skills are foundational in the engaging process and help create a mutual understanding between the counseled and the counselor. Throughout the process, they serve as navigational tools, acting as a guide and catalyst for change.

Open-Ended Questions require elaboration on the part of the counseled individual. They are not readily answered "yes or no." It gives them an opportunity to think a moment before answering and plenty of space to answer. Asking open-ended questions is like opening a door and allowing them to go where they want with it. Asking open-ended questions often yields more information, and more important information than asking a list of predetermined closed questions. *Affirmations* are statements of support that help them identify and reinforce their own strengths. Affirmations must be genuine to build a rapport and to help build their self-confidence in quitting. For example, if you are with a smoker who has tried to quit but were unsuccessful, they may view that as failure and that failure can affect their confidence about another attempt at quitting. Affirming that their decision to quit again shows a strong level of commitment could help change their perspective. *Reflection* (also called reflective thinking) is one of the fundamental skills of MI. It expresses to the smoker that they are not only being heard, but also being understood. It is also an opportunity for them to hear again the feelings and thoughts they are expressing in different words. If reflective listening is effective, it tends to keep them talking and exploring their thoughts and feelings. *Summary*, for the most part, is composed of reflections. The summary recaps many things already discussed during the MI session. The summary simply conveys the point that "I heard you and I understand how it all fits together." This helps continue to build rapport and trust.

8.9 Nicotine Replacement Therapy

The purpose of NRT is to replace much of the nicotine a smoker would obtain from a cigarette, thus reducing their urge to smoke and the nicotine withdrawal symptoms. There are several available delivery methods for NRT: gum, lozenges, inhaler, and patches. The nicotine patch is a transdermal patch placed on a hairless area on the skin.

The nicotine is absorbed through the skin. The patch should be placed in an area above the waist and changed every 24 hours. To avoid skin irritation, rotate the location of placement when changing the patch. The absorption of nicotine through the patch is slower than other NRT products. Also, unlike other products, the absorption is passive and does not mimic any of the behaviors of smoking. Nicotine patches can be purchased over the counter with no prescription required. Nicotine lozenges and gum are also available for purchase over the counter without a prescription. They release nicotine, which is then absorbed through the oral mucosa. These methods are sometimes preferred over the patch because the individual can control the dose of nicotine. One important point to teach smokers trying to quit about the gum is that they should not chew it like regular gum. They should chew it until they feel a bit of a tingle and then park it between their own gum and cheek. This will allow the nicotine to be absorbed. The nicotine inhaler and nasal spray cannot be purchased over the counter. Both require a prescription. The term nicotine inhaler is misleading, given that it does not work the same as an inhaler one would use for asthma where the medication is inhaled into the lungs. The inhaler acts more like a puffer and the medication is absorbed through the oral mucosa and not absorbed through the lungs. The inhaler may be helpful to those who need to replace the sensation of having a cigarette in their mouth. The inhaler is quick acting and takes about the same time to act as the gum. The nasal spray delivers nicotine quickly as it is rapidly absorbed through the nose. It relieves withdrawal symptoms fast, but can be irritating to the nasal passages.

8.10 Medications

Two non-nicotine medications that can be prescribed as stand-alone treatment or in conjunction with NRT to aid an individual in quitting smoking include bupropion SR and varenicline. Evidence has shown when these medications are combined with NRT and counseling, the likelihood of an individual quitting is increased. Bupropion and varenicline are prescribed under the trade names Zyban® and Chantix®, respectively. Varenicline acts on the same receptor site in the brain that nicotine affects. Bupropion blocks the reuptake of dopamine and to a lesser degree, norepinephrine. Therefore, bupropion increases the level of dopamine and norepinephrine. Side effects such as change in behavior, depressed mood, and suicidal thoughts are possible with these medications and individuals need to be educated about the possibility of these side effects and monitored for such.

Suggested Readings

[1] ACOG Committee Opinion No. ACOG Committee Opinion No. 423: motivational interviewing: a tool for behavioral change. Obstet Gynecol. 2009; 113(1):243–246

[2] American College of Radiology. ACR lung cancer screening center. Available at: http://www.acr.org/Quality-Safety/Lung-Cancer-Screening-Center

[3] U.S. Department of Health & Human Services. Get on the Path to a Healthier You. Available at: https://betobaccofree.hhs.gov/gallery/quit-infographic-text.html. Accessed February 02, 2017

[4] Benowitz NL. Neurobiology of nicotine addiction: implications for smoking cessation treatment. Am J Med. 2008; 121(4) Suppl 1:S3–S10

[5] Brown MS, Lo P, Goldin JG, et al. Toward clinically usable CAD for lung cancer screening with computed tomography. Eur Radiol. 2014; 24(11):2719–2728

[6] American Cancer Society. Cancer facts and figures. 2014. Available at:http://www.cancer.org/acs/groups/content/@research/documents/webcontent/acspc-042151.pdf

[7] Cahill K, Stevens S, Perera R, Lancaster T. Pharmacological interventions for smoking cessation: an overview and network meta-analysis. Cochrane Database Syst Rev. 2013(5):CD009329

[8] Centers for Medicare & Medicaid Services. Decision memo for screening for lung cancer with low dose computed tomography (LDCT). (CAG-00439N). Available at: http://www.cms.gov/medicare-coverage-database/details/nca-decision-memo.aspx?NCAId=274

[9] Edwards JP, Datta I, Hunt JD, et al. The impact of computed tomographic screening for lung cancer on the thoracic surgery workforce. Ann Thorac Surg. 2014; 98(2):447–452

[10] Food and Drug Administration. FDA 101: Smoking Cessation Products. 2015. Available at: http://www.fda.gov/ForConsumers/ConsumerUpdates/ucm198176.htm#learn. Accessed January 30, 2017

[11] Donnelly EF. Technical parameters and interpretive issues in screening computed tomography scans for lung cancer. J Thorac Imaging. 2012; 27(4):224–229

[12] U.S. Department of Labor. FAQs about Affordable Care Act Implementation, part XII. Available at: http://www.dol.gov/ebsa/faqs/faq-aca12.html

[13] Fintelmann FJ, Bernheim A, Digumarthy SR, et al. The 10 pillars of lung cancer screening: rationale and logistics of a lung cancer screening program. Radiographics. 2015; 35(7):1893–1908

[14] Gietema HA, Wang Y, Xu D, et al. Pulmonary nodules detected at lung cancer screening: interobserver variability of semiautomated volume measurements. Radiology. 2006; 241(1):251–257

[15] Gomez MM, LoBiondo-Wood G. Lung cancer screening with low-dose CT: its effect on smoking behavior. J Adv Pract Oncol. 2013; 4(6):405–414

[16] American Cancer Society. Guide to quitting smoking. Available at: http://www.cancer.org/healthy/stayawayfromtobacco/guidetoquittingsmoking/index

[17] Centers for Disease Control and Prevention. Health Effects of Cigarette Smoking. 2016. Available at: https://www.cdc.gov/tobacco/data_statistics/fact_sheets/health_effects/effects_cig_smoking/. Accessed February 2, 2017

[18] Centers for Disease Control and Prevention. How to quit. Available at: http://www.cdc.gov/tobacco/quit_smoking/how_to_quit/index.htm

[19] American Lung Association. How to quit smoking. Available at: http://www.lung.org/stop-smoking/how-to-quit/

[20] Horeweg N, van Rosmalen J, Heuvelmans MA, et al. Lung cancer probability in patients with CT-detected pulmonary nodules: a prespecified analysis of data from the NELSON trial of low-dose CT screening. Lancet Oncol. 2014; 15(12):1332–1341

[21] Jeon KN, Goo JM, Lee CH, et al. Computer-aided nodule detection and volumetry to reduce variability between radiologists in the interpretation of lung nodules at low-dose screening computed tomography. Invest Radiol. 2012; 47(8):457–461

[22] Kazerooni EA, Austin JH, Black WC, et al. American College of Radiology, Society of Thoracic Radiology. ACR-STR practice parameter for the performance and reporting of lung cancer screening thoracic computed tomography (CT): 2014 (Resolution 4). J Thorac Imaging. 2014; 29(5):310–316

[23] Kazerooni EA, Armstrong MR, Amorosa JK, et al. ACR CT accreditation program and the lung cancer screening program designation. J Am Coll Radiol. 2015; 12(1):38–42

[24] American College of Radiology. Lung Cancer Screening Resources. Available at: http://www.acr.org/Quality-Safety/Resources/Lung-Imaging-Resources

[25] American Association of Physicists in Medicine. Lung Cancer Screening Protocols. Available at: http://www.aapm.org/pubs/CTProtocols/documents/LungCancerScreeningCT.pdf

[26] American College of Radiology. Lung cancer screening registry. Available at: http://www.acr.org/Quality-Safety/National-Radiology-Data-Registry/Lung-Cancer-Screening-Registry

[27] Martin LJ, Zieve D, Ogilvie I; A.D.A.M. Editorial Ream. Nicotine Replacement Therapy. Available at: https://medlineplus.gov/ency/article/007438.htm. Accessed February 2, 2017

[28] Mazzone P, Powell CA, Arenberg D, et al. Components necessary for high-quality lung cancer screening: American College of Chest Physicians and American Thoracic Society Policy Statement. Chest. 2015; 147(2):295–303

[29] McKee BJ, McKee AB, Kitts AB, Regis SM, Wald C. Low-dose computed tomography screening for lung cancer in a clinical setting: essential elements of a screening program. J Thorac Imaging. 2015; 30(2):115–129

[30] Miller WR, Rollnick S. Motivational Interviewing: Helping People Change. New York, NY: Guilford Press; 2013

[31] Aberle DR, Adams AM, Berg CD, et al. National Lung Screening Trial Research Team. Reduced lung-cancer mortality with low-dose computed tomographic screening. N Engl J Med. 2011; 365(5):395–409

[32] National Comprehensive Cancer Network. NCCN Guidelines for Patients: Lung Cancer Screening. Available at: http://www.nccn.org/patients/guidelines/lung_screening/index.html

[33] American Cancer Society. Nicotine Replacement Therapy for Quitting Tobacco. 2016. Available at: https://www.cancer.org/healthy/stay-away-from-tobacco/guide-quitting-smoking/nicotine-replacement-therapy.html. Accessed February 02, 2017

[34] Parker MS, Groves RC, Fowler AA, III, et al. Lung cancer screening with low-dose computed tomography: an analysis of the MEDCAC decision. J Thorac Imaging. 2015; 30(1):15–23

[35] American Lung Association. Screening for Lung Cancer. Available at: http://www.lung.org/lung-disease/lung-cancer/learning-more-about-lung-cancer/diagnosing-lung-cancer/screening-for-lung-cancer.html

[36] Stead LF, Koilpillai P, Fanshawe TR, Lancaster T. Combined pharmacotherapy and behavioural interventions for smoking cessation. Cochrane Database Syst Rev. 2016; 3(3):CD008286

[37] Stead LF, Perera R, Bullen C, et al. Nicotine replacement therapy for smoking cessation. Cochrane Database Syst Rev. 2012; 11(11):CD000146

[38] Tammemägi MC, Berg CD, Riley TL, Cunningham CR, Taylor KL. Impact of lung cancer screening results on smoking cessation. J Natl Cancer Inst. 2014; 106(6):dju084

[39] National Comprehensive Cancer Network. Quitting smoking for cancer survivors. Available at: http://www.nccn.org/patients/resources/survivorship/smoking.aspx

[40] Villanti AC, Jiang Y, Abrams DB, Pyenson BS. A cost-utility analysis of lung cancer screening and the additional benefits of incorporating smoking cessation interventions. PLoS One. 2013; 8(8):e71379

[41] Centers for Disease Control and Prevention. What Are the Risk Factors for Lung Cancer? 2016. Available at: https://www.cdc.gov/cancer/lung/basic_info/risk_factors.htm. Accessed February 02, 2017

9 Future of Lung Cancer Screening

Samira Shojaee and Deepankar Sharma

Summary

This chapter explores several diverse factors that may potentially predispose different populations to an increased risk of lung cancer including genetic predisposition, dietary habits, cultural beliefs, and environmental exposures. Disparate variations in the detection, diagnosis, staging, and treatment of lung cancer among various ethnic groups and races are also reviewed. The role of various exhaled and serum biomarkers in the early detection, staging, and stratification of lung cancer patients is also discussed and they are likely to have a more prevalent role in the near future to both help identify high-risk populations and minimize false-positive screening rates. Lastly, this chapter reviews various clinical risk assessment models including the Bach, Spitz, LLP (Liverpool Lung Project), and PLCO (Prostate, Lung, Colorectal, and Ovarian) models and demonstrates the application of the Brock University risk calculator.

Keywords: racial disparity, ethnic disparity, epidermal growth factor receptor mutations, oncogenic driver mutation, MicroRNAs, COSMOS, C-reactive protein, prolactin, hepatocyte growth factor, cancer-testis antigen NY-ESO-1, zyxin, osteopontin, ProGRP, S100B, exhaled breath condensate, TNF-α, vascular endothelial growth factor, sICAM-1, bronchial genomic classifier, risk assessment models, Bach model, CARET, Spitz model, Liverpool Lung Project in Liverpool model, Prostate, Lung, Colorectal and Ovarian model, Brock University calculator

9.1 Other Potential Increased Risk Populations

Cigarette smoking is the single most important risk factor for developing lung cancer. Despite the strong relationship between smoking and lung cancer, only about 20% of smokers develop lung cancer. Additionally, about 15 to 25% of new lung cancer diagnoses are in never smokers. Clearly other factors must also play a role in the eventual development of lung cancer.

Diverse factors such as genetic predisposition, dietary habits, cultural beliefs or faith, and environmental exposures have been investigated. Most of these factors overlap and many are common in people of the same race/ethnicity. As such, there has been significant interest in identifying racial differences and susceptibility factors to lung cancer that may affect treatment choice, treatment response, long-term follow-up, and end-of-life care.

In the NLST, 89.6% of the participants were Caucasian, whereas 4% were African Americans and 5% were of other racial groups. About 0.4% had missing racial data. Compared with Caucasians, African Americans tended to be current smokers (albeit less consumption), younger, unmarried, experienced more comorbidity, and had less formal education. However, lung cancer screening (LCS) with low-dose computed tomography (LDCT) was beneficial in all racial groups, resulting in a reduction of lung cancer mortality across all groups, but especially in African Americans. The NLST data also showed that among all racial groups, current smokers had a worse lung cancer–specific mortality, but this risk was **2X** greater in current African American smokers than in Caucasians. Additionally, all-cause mortality was **1.35 times** higher in African

Americans than in Caucasians, but screening with LDCT had a more significant reduction in all-cause mortality in African Americans compared with Caucasians.

Smith et al examined lung cancer stage, treatment, and survival in American Indians and Alaskan Natives. The investigators found these two ethnic groups were more likely to be diagnosed with stage IIIA lung cancer and had lower 5-year survival compared to Caucasians, African Americans, and Hispanics. Racial disparity not only exists in the distribution of lung cancer, but also in treatment choices, hospice utilization, and participation in cancer clinical trials. African American and American Indians are less likely to receive stage-appropriate therapy. Byrne et al demonstrated that even though African Americans and Hispanics were equally willing to participate, Hispanics were less likely to engage in clinical trials due to language barriers, mistrust, and lack of knowledge of clinical trials. Individuals living in areas with a high percentage of either African American or Hispanics were also less likely to use hospice during the 12 months before dying of lung cancer.

Multiple risk factors including economic, behavioral, cultural, genetic, occupational, education, and awareness about screening methods may contribute to disparity in lung cancer incidence, stage at presentation, treatment choices, and survival. Genomic differences also contribute and may explain the racial differences in non–small cell lung cancer (NSCLC). The estimated prevalence of epidermal growth factor receptor (EGFR) mutations in Asians with lung adenocarcinoma is about 50 to 60%, whereas it occurs in only 15 to 20% of Caucasians. There is limited information about oncogenic drivers in African Americans and Hispanics. Steuer et al found that 81% of Asians, 53% of African Americans, and 68% of Hispanics with lung adenocarcinoma had at least one oncogenic driver mutation. Multiple studies have also identified various single nucleotide polymorphisms in Chinese, North Indian, and African American populations. These findings have been linked to an increased incidence of lung cancer along with environmental exposures and by using various prediction models have been used to identify persons at higher risk of lung cancer. Lin et al showed in a study of over 300 persons with lung cancer that African Americans were less likely to receive stage-appropriate therapy compared with Caucasians, even after adjusting for age, sex, marital status, insurance, income, and performance status. These findings were directly related to personal patient beliefs regarding lung cancer, fatalism, and medical distrust. Similar findings were found in both the American Indian and Native Alaskan population. These studies highlight factors other than genetic predisposition, and health care access may explain differences in preference and barriers to receiving stage-appropriate therapy. Hispanics are the largest and fastest growing minority group in the United States and accounted for 17% of U.S. population in 2014. Heterogeneity in lung cancer rates in Hispanics was postulated to reflect smoking patterns and their overall susceptibility to lung cancer. So it may come as a surprise that the overall percentage of Hispanic smokers is actually lower than that observed in both Caucasians and African Americans. Actually the rates are higher among U.S.-born Hispanics than among foreign-born Hispanics. Also, Cubans and Puerto Ricans are more likely to smoke than Mexicans. But, even given similar smoking patterns, Hispanics have a 30 to 70% lower relative risk of developing lung cancer than comparable African American cohorts. Interestingly, EGFR mutations are more common in Hispanics with lung adenocarcinoma than in Caucasians. Furthermore, EGFR mutations are most prevalent in Hispanics from Peru, followed by Costa Rica, Mexico, Panama, Colombia, and Argentina. There are few factors stratifying the risk at a broader level within people of different countries or race. A Chinese population-based study found the risk of lung cancer was higher in nonsmoking persons with a family history of lung cancer or any other cancer.

Dietary factors have also been shown to effect lung cancer development. In one study, higher intake of carbohydrates and fiber and lower intake of animal fat and protein have a protective effect against lung cancer. However, when adjusted for smoking history, these dietary effects were not statistically significant. This finding is consistent with recommendations of the American Institute for Cancer Research that report carotenoid containing fruits along with nonstarchy vegetables have a protective effect against lung cancer. There is limited evidence suggesting red meat, total fat intake, and processed meat increase the risk of lung cancer. Dietary factors are often influenced by geography, ethnicity, and country of origin and can indirectly explain the racial disparity and populations at higher risk for lung cancer.

More than 11% of the U.S. population is foreign born. Immigrant population is a higher risk population due to underrepresentation in cancer-related data collection and involvement in National Cancer Institute (NCI) sponsored clinical trials. Immigrants with limited English proficiency risk being excluded from cancer research. Later stage diagnoses and higher mortality suggests that cancer disparities are common in immigrant populations. Another possible reason for such underrepresentation may be a return to the country of origin by those immigrants who wish to spend their final days among family.

Populations with chronic lung disease are also at higher risk for lung cancer. Chronic inflammation associated with diseases like chronic obstructive pulmonary disease (COPD), asthma, and tuberculosis has been contemplated to be the underlying reason for the increased risk of lung cancer in these individuals.

Islami et al even further illustrate the racial and geographic disparity in incidence, prevalence, and mortality of lung cancer. By examining age-standardized lung cancer death rates by education, race, and ethnicity, these authors concluded that 73% of U.S. lung cancer deaths could be prevented each year if overall population rates were reduced to those of educated Caucasians in lower risk states.

9.2 Role of Biomarkers

In the absence of LCS with LDCT, more than 75% of lung cancers currently will not be diagnosed until after the disease is already locally advanced or has metastasized resulting in such dismal survival rates. The 5-year survival rate in stage I NSCLC is approximately 50 to 70%. In contrast, the 5-year survival rate drops to 5 to 15% and less than 2% for patients with stage III and IV NSCLC, respectively. Obviously, diagnosing lung cancer at its earliest stages will effectively reduce mortality. Biomarkers will likely have a more prevalent role in the near future to help identify both high-risk populations while keeping false-positive rates to minimum.

Many such biomarkers have been studied and are being developed for this specific purpose. **MicroRNAs** (miRNAs) are one such class of biomarkers. These small, highly conversed noncoding RNAs are involved in many developmental processes and act as posttranscriptional regulators of gene expression. **miRNAs** regulate many biologic processes, including differentiation, proliferation, and apoptosis. Altered **miRNAs** expression is associated with various human cancers, acting instead as oncogenes or tumor suppressor genes. Wang et al developed a panel of three **miRNAs** identified in the serum of patients with early- and advanced-stage lung cancer using the TaqMan probe–based real-time reverse transcription quantitative polymerase chain reaction (RT-qPCR). These three **miRNAs** (miR-125a-5p, miR-25, and miR-126) were capable of distinguishing early-stage lung cancer patients from controls with 87.5% sensitivity and 87.5% specificity, respectively. Montani et al developed a panel of 13 **miRNAs** and performed a large-scale validation study in 1,115 high-risk individuals enrolled in the Continuous Observation of Smoking Subjects (COSMOS) LCS program. The overall accuracy, sensitivity, and specificity of the **miRNA test** are 74.9, 77.8, and 74.8%, respectively. Sestini et al demonstrated that a 24-plasma-based microRNA signature classifier (MSC) was capable of increasing the specificity of LDCT in a LCS trial. Five-year survival was 88.9% for low-risk MSC, 79.5% for intermediate-risk MSC, and 40.1% for high-risk MSC. The prognostic power of MSC persisted after adjusting for tumor stage. The results from a study by Li et al suggested that miR-486 and miR-150 could serve as potential blood-based biomarkers for the early diagnosis of NSCLC. Monitoring changes in miR-486 expression in plasma might be an effective method for predicting recurrence in early-staged NSCLC patients.

Ma et al tested a panel of four serum proteins: **C-reactive protein (CRP)**, **prolactin**, **hepatocyte growth factor (HGF)**, and **circulating autoantibody against cancer-testis antigen NY-ESO-1**. Using the concentrations of all four markers as a panel along with age, gender, and smoking status, the adjusted prediction model correctly discriminated patients with benign nodules from those with lung cancer with 86.96% sensitivity and 98.25% specificity.

Kim et al detected a total of 17 proteins that were significantly elevated in the plasma of NSCLC patients, which could represent potential tumor markers. One of the novel plasma-based tumor markers, **Zyxin**, demonstrated a potential role as an early diagnostic marker for NSCLC.

Osteopontin (OPN) is a multifunctional cytokine involved in carcinogenesis. Kerenidi et al, in a prospective cohort study, showed increased baseline **OPN** circulating levels in lung cancer patients compared with controls. They also found a significant association between serum OPN levels and certain clinical parameters, including smoking status, weight loss, and performance status. In addition, their study demonstrated patients with lower OPN levels had better survival.

The primary goal of biomarkers is to identify lung cancer in its earliest stages. But biomarkers may also aid in differentiating the specific subtype of lung cancer. Yang et al, in their study of four biomarkers, found adding **ProGRP** increased the specificity of a previous panel of tumor markers, such as CEA (carcinoembryonic antigen), SCC, and CYFRA21–1, for NSCLC from 89.1 to 100%. Therefore, **ProGRP** could potentially help differentiate SCLC from NSCLC and obviate misdiagnosis of the former. Similarly, Choi et al demonstrated the role of serum **S100B** and **S100B autoantibodies** to identify brain metastasis in patients with lung cancer. This is based on the underlying principle that **S100B** is an astrocytic protein that enters the blood stream only when there is disruption of the blood–brain barrier (BBB). Over time, antibodies against S100B develop in the sera of patients with persistent or repeated BBB violations.

Exhaled breath condensate (EBC) is an area of great interest to many investigators. Cheng and colleagues found the expression of keratins 14, 16, and 17 was significantly different between the **EBC** of patients with NSCLC and healthy controls. It is unknown at this time whether these keratins are derived from the airways or from ambient air. Due to large variations in the levels of keratin expression in the respiratory tract between individuals, their use for diagnostic purposes is not recommended as a stand-alone biomarker at this time.

Cytokines in EBC have been widely studied targeting the detection of IL-6, vascular endothelial growth factor (VEGF), TNF-α, IL-8, and soluble intercellular adhesion molecule-1 (siCAM1). Carpagnano et al first detected increased **levels** of *EBC IL-6* in NSCLC patients compared with controls and reported a significant positive correlation between *IL-6* levels and increasing disease stage. Brussino et al showed that increased *EBC IL-6* (along with IL-17 and TNF-α) was associated with increased levels of *EBC VEGF*, and all of these biomarkers correlated significantly with tumor diameter. Dalaveris et al also reported increased *TNF-α* and *VEGF* in patients with stages III and IV NSCLC. In another study by Carpagnano et al, increased levels of *EBC IL-2*, *TNF-α*, and *leptin* were found in patients with stages I and II NSCLC compared with healthy former smokers. Jungraithmayr et al reported *EBC* and preoperative levels of *TNF-α* and *sICAM-1* were significantly higher in bronchial carcinoma compared with controls undergoing thoracoscopy with minimal wedge resection. Kullmann et al published one of the few studies using a multiplexed proteomic approach to study EBC in lung cancer. These authors showed the cytokine profile in EBC of lung cancer patients was different from that of controls, regardless of their smoking habits, lung function, and airway inflammation.

Using *exhaled biomarkers* could be an ideal screening tool for the early detection of lung cancer because *EBC* collection is safe, noninvasive, and can be easily repeated. Moreover, *EBC biomarkers* closely represent the respiratory milieu, which could reveal subtle changes in the airway due to pathogenesis and is ideal for screening of early-stage disease in high-risk populations. However, it is not yet known if exhaled biomarkers will reveal disease-induced variations earlier or prove to be more sensitive compared to traditional systemic markers (e.g., serum and plasma) and/or imaging techniques (e.g., LDCT). Before *EBC* can be more broadly tested clinically, refinement of breath collection and processing methods is critical. Further studies improving the efficacy of breath condensers and standardization of EBC sampling and protein determination are required.

Bronchial genomic classifier is one of few biomarker assays commercially available. Its potential role was demonstrated in the Airway Epithelium Gene Expression in the Diagnosis of Lung Cancer (AEGIS) trials (AEGIS-1 and AEGIS-2) that enrolled 639 total patients. In these trials, 43% of bronchoscopic examinations were nondiagnostic for lung cancer, and invasive procedures were performed after bronchoscopy in 35% of patients with benign lesions. In AEGIS-1, the classifier had a sensitivity of 88% and a specificity of 47%. In AEGIS-2, the classifier had a sensitivity of 89% and a specificity of 47%. The combination of the classifier plus bronchoscopy increased sensitivity to 98% in AEGIS-2, independent of both lesion size and location. The gene-expression classifier improved the diagnostic performance of bronchoscopy for the detection of lung cancer. In intermediate-risk patients with a nondiagnostic bronchoscopic examination, a negative classifier score provided support for a more conservative diagnostic approach. A follow-up study to determine the clinical implication of these results suggested recommendations for invasive procedures were reduced from 57% without the classifier to 18% with a low-risk classifier result. Invasive procedure recommendations increased from 50 to 65% with a positive (intermediate-risk) classifier result. When stratifying by ultimate disease diagnosis, there was an overall reduction in invasive procedure recommendations in patients with benign disease when classifier results were reported (54–41%). For patients ultimately diagnosed with malignant disease, there was an overall increase in invasive procedure recommendations when the classifier results were reported (50–64%).

Salivary microbiota are another class of potential biomarkers. Yan et al showed salivary *Capnocytophaga* and *Veillonella* had an 84.6% sensitivity and 86.7% specificity in distinguishing patients with squamous cell lung cancer from controls and 78.6% sensitivity and 80.0% specificity in distinguishing those with lung adenocarcinoma from controls.

A few in vitro studies have demonstrated other potential biomarkers including *Stanniocalcin-2*. The latter was elevated in tissue samples of patients with lung cancer and seemed to have influential role in the development of metastasis, but this has not been validated in prospective in vivo studies.

9.3 Risk Assessment

Relatively few models have been developed to predict lung cancer risk. One of the oldest models was the Harvard Cancer Risk Index. This model relied on risk estimates from the literature and group consensus. In the past decade, three more sophisticated absolute risk models have been developed. These include the Bach, Spitz, and the Liverpool Lung Project (LLP) models. Although there are some similarities among these three models (e.g., asbestos exposure, duration of smoking), the models do vary to an extent. The differences are primarily based on personal history of malignancy, family history of malignancy, and lung-related comorbidities (emphysema vs. pneumonia). Tammemagi et al also developed and validated another risk prediction tool for current and former smokers and made it applicable to the NLST data.

9.3.1 Bach Model

The Bach model arose from the β-Carotene and Retinol Efficacy Trial (CARET). CARET was a multicenter randomized, controlled study of β-carotene and vitamin A supplementation in over 14,000 heavy smokers (mostly men) and over 4,000 men with asbestos exposure. Using a Cox proportional hazards regression, Bach and colleagues devised a model to assess the 1-year probability of lung cancer diagnosis and the competing risk of dying without lung cancer. Model variables included age, sex, number of cigarettes smoked per day, number of years smoked, number of years quit (former smokers), and asbestos exposure. To obtain 10-year absolute risk estimates for an individual being diagnosed with lung cancer, the 1-year models are run recursively 10 times each to develop a sum of probabilities over time. For each year, the chance of diagnosis is determined by multiplying the person's chance of being diagnosed with lung cancer from the incidence model by the chance that the person is alive in that year. Bach et al presented 10-year absolute risk for lung cancer stating the 10-year absolute risk is perhaps in excess of the time it takes for lung cancer to progress from an undetectable size to an untreatable stage. They also concluded this model was useful in educating patients about the merits of screening.

9.3.2 Spitz Model

The Spitz model is based on 1,851 lung cancer cases and about 2,000 matched controls (age, sex, race, smoking status) from a lung cancer case control study. Spitz and colleagues combined the baseline relative risk from the model, with age- and gender-specific incidence rates corrected for smoking status and all-cause mortality excluding lung cancer to estimate an X-year absolute risk of lung cancer.

9.3.3 LLP Model

The LLP model was created using 579 patients with lung cancer and 1,157 age- and sex-matched population-based controls from a case control study out of the LLP in Liverpool, UK. Using logistic regression, their model estimated lung cancer relative risk. This model was used by Chen et al to combine the relative risk estimates and lung cancer incidence rates and presented as a 5-year absolute lung cancer risk.

9.3.4 Prostate, Lung, Colorectal, and Ovarian Model 2012

Tammemagi et al developed a lung cancer risk prediction model involving former and current smokers in the Prostate, Lung, Colorectal, and Ovarian (PLCO) cancer screening trial control and intervention groups. Predictors used in this model included age, education level, body mass index (BMI), family history of lung cancer, COPD, chest X-ray in the past 3 years, smoking status (current vs. former smoker), pack-years and duration of cigarette smoking, and quit time (i.e., number of years since the person quit). This model showed high predictive discrimination measured with the use of the area under the receiver operating characteristic curve (AUC), but proved cumbersome to apply. Model risks were also based on 9.2 years' median follow-up, which was longer than the NLST, so the estimates were inaccurate when applied to the NLST data. In order to make the risk prediction model directly applicable to NLST collected data, PLCO Model 2012 was developed and validated. This new model was built using logistic regression data from 80,375 persons in the PLCO control and intervention groups who had ever smoked to predict their 6-year risk of lung cancer. The PLCO Model 2012 proved more sensitive than the NLST criteria for lung cancer detection. The AUC was 0.803 in the development data set and 0.797 in the validation data set. As compared with NLST criteria, PLCO Model 2012 criteria had improved sensitivity (83.0 vs. 71.1%, $p < 0.001$) and positive predictive value (4.0 vs. 3.4%, $p = 0.01$), without loss of specificity (62.9 and 62.7%, respectively; $p = 0.54$); 41.3% and fewer lung cancers were missed.

9.3.5 Brock University Calculator

Brock University Calculator (https://brocku.ca/lung-cancer-risk-calculator), one of the most commonly used lung cancer prediction calculators for clinicians, uses the above models for risk calculation. The Brock calculator can be easily utilized in the emergency departments, radiology departments, and outpatient and inpatient setting to estimate an individual's lung cancer risk based on their history and chest imaging. For example, using the Brock calculator, a clinician can estimate a cancer probability of 0.23% in a 73-year-old male patient, smoker with emphysema, no family history of lung cancer with a single 4-mm nonsolid pulmonary nodule. Applying the same prediction model, this risk increases to 0.42% if the person's gender is changed from male to female. The risk increases still further to 0.82%, if the pulmonary nodule is located in the upper lobe. The Brock calculator provides both lung cancer estimates in percentile and the log odds of having cancer. Despite easy use and accessibility, many clinicians remain unfamiliar with Brock University cancer prediction equation. However, risk stratification models or calculators of this nature are likely to have more and more of a prominent role in the near future, streamlining and selecting those at-risk individuals that will most benefit from early-detection LDCT LCS, rather than relying on age and pack-years of smoking alone.

Suggested Readings

[1] Arrieta O, Ramírez-Tirado L-A, Báez-Saldaña R, Peña-Curiel O, Soca-Chafre G, Macedo-Perez E-O. Different mutation profiles and clinical characteristics among Hispanic patients with non-small cell lung cancer could explain the "Hispanic paradox.". Lung Cancer. 2015; 90(2):161–166

[2] Bach PB, Kattan MW, Thornquist MD, et al. Variations in lung cancer risk among smokers. J Natl Cancer Inst. 2003; 95(6):470–478

[3] Brussino L, Culla B, Bucca C, et al. Inflammatory cytokines and VEGF measured in exhaled breath condensate are correlated with tumor mass in non-small cell lung cancer. J Breath Res. 2014; 8(2):027110

[4] Byrne MM, Tannenbaum SL, Glück S, Hurley J, Antoni M. Participation in cancer clinical trials: why are patients not participating? Med Decis Making. 2014; 34(1):116–126

[5] Carpagnano GE, Resta O, Foschino-Barbaro MP, Gramiccioni E, Carpagnano F. Interleukin-6 is increased in breath condensate of patients with non-small cell lung cancer. Int J Biol Markers. 2002; 17(2):141–145

[6] Carpagnano GE, Spanevello A, Curci C, et al. IL-2, TNF-alpha, and leptin: local versus systemic concentrations in NSCLC patients. Oncol Res. 2007; 16(8):375–381

[7] Cheng Y, Jiang T, Zhu M, et al. Risk assessment models for genetic risk predictors of lung cancer using two-stage replication for Asian and European populations. Oncotarget Advance Publications 2016. www.impactjournals.com/oncotarget/. Published July 5, 2016.

[8] Cheng Z, Lewis CR, Thomas PS, Raftery MJ. Comparative proteomics analysis of exhaled breath condensate in lung cancer patients. J Cancer Ther. 2011; 2(1):1–8

[9] Chen J, Pee D, Ayyagari R, et al. Projecting absolute invasive breast cancer risk in white women with a model that includes mammographic density. J Natl Cancer Inst. 2006; 98(17):1215–1226

[10] Choi H, Puvenna V, Brennan C, et al. S100B and S100B autoantibody as biomarkers for early detection of brain metastases in lung cancer. Transl Lung Cancer Res. 2016; 5(4):413–419

[11] Colditz GA, Atwood KA, Emmons K, et al. Harvard report on cancer prevention volume 4: Harvard Cancer Risk Index. Risk Index Working Group, Harvard Center for Cancer Prevention. Cancer Causes Control. 2000; 11(6):477–488

[12] Dalaveris E, Kerenidi T, Katsabeki-Katsafli A, et al. VEGF, TNF-alpha and 8-isoprostane levels in exhaled breath condensate and serum of patients with lung cancer. Lung Cancer. 2009; 64(2):219–225

[13] Dominguez K, Penman-Aguilar A, Chang M-H, et al. Centers for Disease Control and Prevention (CDC). Vital signs: leading causes of death, prevalence of diseases and risk factors, and use of health services among Hispanics in the United States—2009–2013. MMWR Morb Mortal Wkly Rep. 2015; 64(17):469–478

[14] Ferguson JS, Van Wert R, Choi Y, et al. Impact of a bronchial genomic classifier on clinical decision making in patients undergoing diagnostic evaluation for lung cancer. BMC Pulm Med. 2016; 16(1):66

[15] Ferlay J, Shin H-R, Bray F, Forman D, Mathers C, Parkin DM. Estimates of worldwide burden of cancer in 2008: GLOBOCAN 2008. Int J Cancer. 2010; 127(12):2893–2917

[16] Fontana RS, Sanderson DR, Woolner LB, et al. Screening for lung cancer. A critique of the Mayo Lung Project. Cancer. 1991; 67(4) Suppl:1155–1164

[17] Gany FM, Shah SM, Changrani J. New York City's immigrant minorities. Reducing cancer health disparities. Cancer. 2006; 107(8) Suppl:2071–2081

[18] Glade MJ. Food, nutrition, and the prevention of cancer: a global perspective. American Institute for Cancer Research/World Cancer Research Fund, American Institute for Cancer Research, 1997. Nutrition. 1999; 15(6):523–526

[19] Gould MK, Tang T, Liu I-LA, et al. Recent trends in the identification of incidental pulmonary nodules. Am J Respir Crit Care Med. 2015; 192(10):1208–1214

[20] Haas JS, Earle CC, Orav JE, et al. Lower use of hospice by cancer patients who live in minority versus white areas. J Gen Intern Med. 2007; 22(3):396–399

[21] Haiman CA, Stram DO, Wilkens LR, et al. Ethnic and racial differences in the smoking-related risk of lung cancer. N Engl J Med. 2006; 354(4):333–342

[22] Hayes SA, Haefliger S, Harris B, et al. Exhaled breath condensate for lung cancer protein analysis: a review of methods and biomarkers. J Breath Res. 2016; 10(3):034001

[23] Heller G, Weinzierl M, Noll C, et al. Genome-wide miRNA expression profiling identifies miR-9-3 and miR-193a as targets for DNA methylation in non-small cell lung cancers. Clin Cancer Res. 2012; 18(6):1619–1629

[24] Huang J-Y, Jian Z-H, Nfor ON, et al. The effects of pulmonary diseases on histologic types of lung cancer in both sexes: a population-based study in Taiwan. BMC Cancer. 2015; 15:834

[25] Ihsan R, Chauhan PS, Mishra AK, et al. Copy number polymorphism of glutathione-S-transferase genes (GSTM1 & GSTT1) in susceptibility to lung cancer in a high-risk population from north-east India. Indian J Med Res. 2014; 139(5):720–729

[26] Islami F, Ward EM, Jacobs EJ, et al. Potentially preventable premature lung cancer deaths in the USA if overall population rates were reduced to those of educated whites in lower-risk states. Cancer Causes Control. 2015; 26(3):409–418

[27] Jamal A, Homa DM, O'Connor E, et al. Current cigarette smoking among adults - United States, 2005–2014. MMWR Morb Mortal Wkly Rep. 2015; 64(44):1233–1240

[28] Jungraithmayr W, Frings C, Zissel G, Prasse A, Passlick B, Stoelben E. Inflammatory markers in exhaled breath condensate following lung resection for bronchial carcinoma. Respirology. 2008; 13(7):1022–1027

[29] Kaplan RC, Bangdiwala SI, Barnhart JM, et al. Smoking among U.S. Hispanic/Latino adults: the Hispanic community health study/study of Latinos. Am J Prev Med. 2014; 46(5):496–506

[30] Koukiidl T, Kazakou AP, Lada M, Tsilioni I, Daniil Z, Gourgoulianis KI. Clinical significance of circulating osteopontin levels in patients with lung cancer and correlation with VEGF and MMP-9. Cancer Invest. 2016; 34(8):385–392

[31] Kim YJ, Sertamo K, Pierrard M-A, et al. Verification of the biomarker candidates for non-small-cell lung cancer using a targeted proteomics approach. J Proteome Res. 2015; 14(3):1412–1419

[32] Landi MT, Zhao Y, Rotunno M, et al. MicroRNA expression differentiates histology and predicts survival of lung cancer. Clin Cancer Res. 2010; 16(2):430–441

[33] Li W, Wang Y, Zhang Q, et al. MicroRNA-486 as a biomarker for early diagnosis and recurrence of non-small cell lung cancer. PLoS One. 2015; 10(8):e0134220

[34] Lin H, Huang Y-S, Yan HH, et al. A family history of cancer and lung cancer risk in never-smokers: a clinic-based case-control study. Lung Cancer. 2015; 89(2):94–98

[35] Lin JJ, Mhango G, Wall MM, et al. Cultural factors associated with racial disparities in lung cancer care. Ann Am Thorac Soc. 2014; 11(4):489–495

[36] Lin P-Y, Yang P-C. Circulating miRNA signature for early diagnosis of lung cancer. EMBO Mol Med. 2011; 3 (8):436–437

[37] Little AG, Gay EG, Gaspar LE, Stewart AK. National survey of non-small cell lung cancer in the United States: epidemiology, pathology and patterns of care. Lung Cancer. 2007; 57(3):253–260

[38] Ma S, Wang W, Xia B, et al. Multiplexed serum biomarkers for the detection of lung cancer. EBioMedicine. 2016; 11:210–218

[39] Machiela MJ, Hsiung CA, Shu X-O, et al. Genetic variants associated with longer telomere length are associated with increased lung cancer risk among never-smoking women in Asia: a report from the female lung cancer consortium in Asia. Int J Cancer. 2015; 137(2):311–319

[40] Montani F, Marzi MJ, Dezi F, et al. miR-Test: a blood test for lung cancer early detection. J Natl Cancer Inst. 2015; 107(6):djv063

[41] Na SS, Aldonza MB, Sung H-J, et al. Stanniocalcin-2 (STC2): a potential lung cancer biomarker promotes lung cancer metastasis and progression. Biochim Biophys Acta. 2015; 1854(6):668–676

[42] Aberle DR, Adams AM, Berg CD, et al. National Lung Screening Trial Research Team. Reduced lung-cancer mortality with low-dose computed tomographic screening. N Engl J Med. 2011; 365(5):395–409

[43] National Cancer Institute. SEER Cancer Stat Facts: Lung and Bronchus Cancer. Bethesda, MD: National Cancer Institute; 2015

[44] Redova M, Sana J, Slaby O. Circulating miRNAs as new blood-based biomarkers for solid cancers. Future Oncol. 2013; 9(3):387–402

[45] Saito M, Schetter AJ, Mollerup S, et al. The association of microRNA expression with prognosis and progression in early-stage, non-small cell lung adenocarcinoma: a retrospective analysis of three cohorts. Clin Cancer Res. 2011; 17(7):1875–1882

[46] Sestini S, Boeri M, Marchiano A, et al. Circulating microRNA signature as liquid-biopsy to monitor lung cancer in low-dose computed tomography screening. Oncotarget. 2015; 6(32):32868–32877

[47] Sharma N, Singh A, Singh N, Behera D, Sharma S. Genetic polymorphisms in GSTM1, GSTT1 and GSTP1 genes and risk of lung cancer in a North Indian population. Cancer Epidemiol. 2015; 39(6):947–955

[48] Shen W, Yin R, Wang C, et al. Polymorphisms in alternative splicing associated genes are associated with lung cancer risk in a Chinese population. Lung Cancer. 2015; 89(3):238–242

[49] Silvestri GA, Vachani A, Whitney D, et al. AEGIS Study Team. A bronchial genomic classifier for the diagnostic evaluation of lung cancer. N Engl J Med. 2015; 373(3):243–251

[50] Smith CB, Bonomi M, Packer S, Wisnivesky JP. Disparities in lung cancer stage, treatment and survival among American Indians and Alaskan Natives. Lung Cancer. 2011; 72(2):160–164

[51] Spitz MR, Hong WK, Amos CI, et al. A risk model for prediction of lung cancer. J Natl Cancer Inst. 2007; 99(9): 715–726

[52] Steuer CE, Behera M, Berry L, et al. Role of race in oncogenic driver prevalence and outcomes in lung adenocarcinoma: results from the Lung Cancer Mutation Consortium. Cancer. 2016; 122(5):766–772

[53] Stern MC, Fejerman L, Das R, et al. Variability in cancer risk and outcomes within US Latinos by national origin and genetic ancestry. Curr Epidemiol Rep. 2016; 3:181–190

[54] Tammemägi MC, Katki HA, Hocking WG, et al. Selection criteria for lung-cancer screening. N Engl J Med. 2013; 368(8):728–736

[55] Tammemagi CM, Pinsky PF, Caporaso NE, et al. Lung cancer risk prediction: Prostate, Lung, Colorectal and Ovarian Cancer Screening Trial models and validation. J Natl Cancer Inst. 2011; 103(13):1058–1068

[56] Tanner NT, Gebregziabher M, Hughes Halbert C, Payne E, Egede LE, Silvestri GA. Racial differences in outcomes within the national lung screening trial. implications for widespread implementation. Am J Respir Crit Care Med. 2015; 192(2):200–208

[57] Tanoue LT, Tanner NT, Gould MK, Silvestri GA. Lung cancer screening. Am J Respir Crit Care Med. 2015; 191 (1):19–33

[58] Tsai Y-Y, McGlynn KA, Hu Y, et al. Genetic susceptibility and dietary patterns in lung cancer. Lung Cancer. 2003; 41(3):269–281

[59] Wang P, Yang D, Zhang H, et al. Early detection of lung cancer in serum by a panel of MicroRNA biomarkers. Clin Lung Cancer. 2015; 16(4):313–31–9.e1

[60] Yan X, Yang M, Liu J, et al. Discovery and validation of potential bacterial biomarkers for lung cancer. Am J Cancer Res. 2015; 5(10):3111–3122

[61] Yang D-W, Zhang Y, Hong Q-Y, et al. Role of a serum-based biomarker panel in the early diagnosis of lung cancer for a cohort of high-risk patients. Cancer. 2015; 121 Suppl 17:3113–3121

[62] Zanetti KA, Wang Z, Aldrich M, et al. Genome-wide association study confirms lung cancer susceptibility loci on chromosomes 5p15 and 15q25 in an African-American population. Lung Cancer. 2016; 98:33–42

10 Test Cases: Applying Lung CT Screening Reporting and Data System (Lung-RADS)

Mark S. Parker, Leila Rezai Gharai, Joanna E. Kusmirek, and Robert C. Groves

Summary

This final chapter will test your knowledge and application of the Lung CT Screening Reporting and Data System (Lung-RADS). You will be shown 10 unknown cases. For each unknown case, determine the appropriate Lung-RADS score and best course of management. The correct answer(s) will follow.

Keywords: Lung-RADS 1, Lung-RADS 2, Lung-RADS 3, Lung-RADS 4, solid nodule, ground-glass nodule, part-solid nodule, pericystic nodule

10.1 Case 1

Axial low-dose computed tomography (LDCT) screen-selected mediastinal (▶ Fig. 10.1**a**) and lung window (▶ Fig. 10.1**b**) images of an asymptomatic current female smoker demonstrate a 12-mm solid, rounded, soft-tissue attenuation noncalcified endobronchial lesion that nearly occludes the lingular bronchus lumen. What is the correct Lung-RADS category and appropriate course of management?

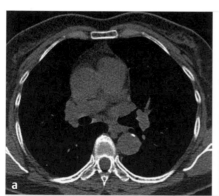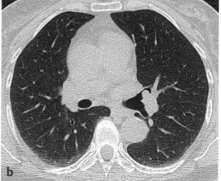

Fig. 10.1 (a) Axial low-dose computed tomography (LDCT) screen-selected mediastinal and (b) lung window images of an asymptomatic current female smoker demonstrates a 12-mm solid, rounded, soft-tissue attenuation noncalcified endobronchial lesion that nearly occludes the lingular bronchus lumen.

10.2 Case 2

Coned-down axial LDCT screen (▶ Fig. 10.2) through the right lower lobe of a 65-year-old woman shows a 7-mm total diameter part-solid nodule composed primarily of ground-glass but with a 3-mm solid component on baseline screening LDCT. What is the correct Lung-RADS category and appropriate course of management?

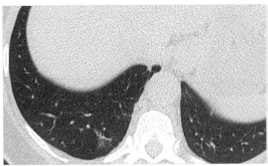

Fig. 10.2 Coned-down axial low-dose computed tomography (LDCT) screen through the right lower lobe of a 65-year-old woman shows a 7-mm total diameter part-solid nodule composed primarily of ground-glass but with a 3-mm solid component on baseline screening LDCT.

10.3 Case 3

Coned-down axial LDCT screen (▶ Fig. 10.3) through the left lower lobe of a current smoking 55-year-old woman reveals a 6.2-mm average diameter solid, spiculated, noncalcified nodule in the superior segment ($5.3 + 7.1 \div 2 = 6.2$ mm) on baseline screening LDCT. The nodule is rounded off to the nearest whole number or 6 mm in diameter. Note the background of extensive centrilobular emphysema (score: 3/3). What is the correct Lung-RADS category and appropriate course of management?

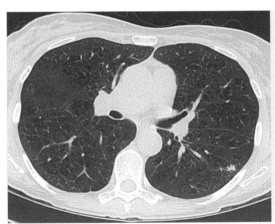

Fig. 10.3 Coned-down axial low-dose computed tomography (LDCT) screen through the left lower lobe of a current smoking 55-year-old woman reveals a 6.2-mm average diameter solid, spiculated, noncalcified nodule in the superior segment ($5.3 + 7.1 \div 2 = 6.2$ mm) on baseline screening LDCT. The nodule is rounded off to the nearest whole number or 6 mm in diameter. Note the background of extensive centrilobular emphysema (score: 3/3).

10.4 Case 4

Coned-down axial LDCT screen (▶ Fig. 10.4) through the posterior segment of the right upper lobe of a 73-year-old woman, current cigarette smoker with a total 43-pack-year history of tobacco abuse, shows a pure ground-glass nodule (GGN) measuring 14 mm in maximum diameter. Although some margins appear slightly irregular, there is no solid component present and there is no architectural distortion. What is the correct Lung-RADS category and appropriate course of management?

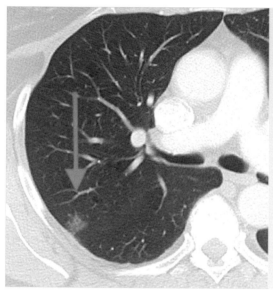

Fig. 10.4 Coned-down axial low-dose computed tomography (LDCT) screen through the posterior segment of the right upper lobe of a 73-year-old female, current cigarette smoker with a total 43-pack-year history of tobacco abuse, shows a pure ground-glass nodule measuring 14 mm in maximum diameter. Although some margins appear slightly irregular, there is no solid component present and there is no architectural distortion.

10.5 Case 5

Baseline LDCT screen (▶ Fig. 10.5a) of a 69-year-old former heavy smoker asymptomatic man demonstrates a 10-mm slightly lobulated nodule with an irregular border superiorly. A 3 month follow-up LDCT was recommended but not performed until 4 months later (▶ Fig. 10.5b), which shows significant interval growth of the lesion to 18 mm with increased polylobulation and spiculated borders. Note the notch at the 7:00 plane. How would you categorize the Lung-RADS score on both the baseline (▶ Fig. 10.5a) and follow-up study (▶ Fig. 10.5b)? What is the appropriate course of management at this time? Calculate the percent growth of this lesion.

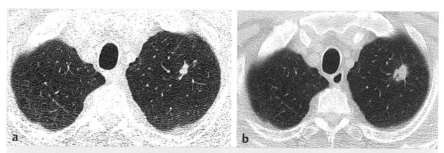

Fig. 10.5 **(a)** Baseline low-dose computed tomography (LDCT) screen of a 69-year-old former heavy smoker asymptomatic man demonstrates a 10-mm slightly lobulated nodule with an irregular border superiorly. **(b)** A 3-month follow-up LDCT was recommended but not performed until 4 months later, which showed significant interval growth of the lesion to 18 mm with increased polylobulation and spiculated borders. Note the notch at the 7 o'clock plane.

10.6 Case 6

Baseline LDCT screen (▶ Fig. 10.6a) of a 69-year-old former heavy smoker asymptomatic woman shows a part-solid pericystic lesion in the peripheral anterior segment of the right upper lobe. The total diameter is 9 mm. Two subtle solid components to the lesion are identified at the 12 o'clock position (▶ Fig. 10.6a). Follow-up LDCT 6 months later (▶ Fig. 10.6b) shows near-complete solid replacement of the cystic component of the lesion. Even though the total diameter is still 9 mm, the solid component has significantly increased and the borders are more polylobulated. How would you categorize the Lung-RADS score on both the baseline (▶ Fig. 10.6a) and follow-up study (▶ Fig. 10.6b)? Do you agree with the initial recommendation to follow up the lesion in question in 6 months? What is the appropriate course of management at this time?

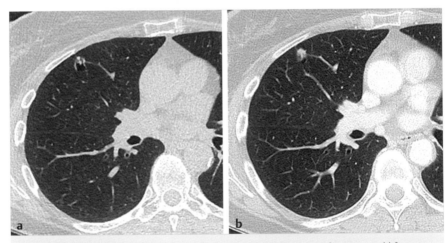

Fig. 10.6 (a) Baseline low-dose computed tomography (LDCT) screen of a 69-year-old former heavy smoker asymptomatic woman shows a part-solid pericystic lesion in the peripheral anterior segment of the right upper lobe. The total diameter is 9 mm. Two subtle solid components to the lesion are identified at the 12 o'clock position. (b) Follow-up LDCT 6 months later shows near-complete solid replacement of the cystic component of the lesion. Even though the total diameter is still 9 mm, the solid component has significantly increased and the borders are more polylobulated.

10.7 Case 7

Coned-down axial LDCT screen (▶ Fig. 10.7) through the superior segment of the right lower lobe of a 60-year-old woman with a history of former heavy tobacco abuse shows an 18-mm solid, noncalcified, polylobulated nodule with spiculated borders on baseline screening LDCT. Note the "notches" at the 2 and 4 o'clock positions. What is the correct Lung-RADS category and appropriate course of management?

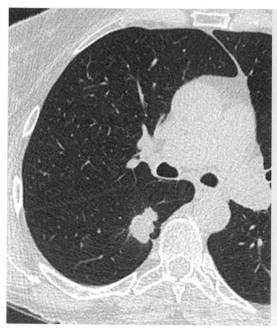

Fig. 10.7 Coned-down axial low-dose computed tomography (LDCT) screen through the superior segment of the right lower lobe of a 60-year-old woman with a history of former heavy tobacco abuse shows an 18-mm solid, noncalcified, polylobulated nodule with spiculated borders on baseline screening LDCT. Note the "notches" at the 2 and 4 o'clock positions.

10.8 Case 8

Coned-down axial LDCT screen (▶ Fig. 10.8) through the right upper lobe of a man with a history of current heavy tobacco abuse and chronic obstructive pulmonary disease (COPD) shows a 7-mm solid, noncalcified rounded nodule in the medial posterior segment of the right upper lobe on a background of moderate emphysema (score: 2/3). What is the correct Lung-RADS category and appropriate course of management?

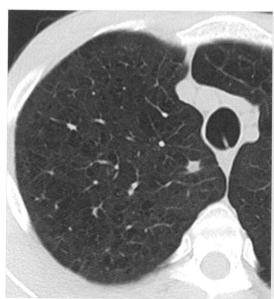

Fig. 10.8 Coned-down axial low-dose computed tomography (LDCT) screen through the right upper lobe of a man with a history of current heavy tobacco abuse and COPD shows a 7-mm solid, noncalcified rounded nodule in the medial posterior segment of the right upper lobe on a background of moderate emphysema (score: 2/3).

10.9 Case 9

Axial LDCT image through the right upper lobe (▶ Fig. 10.9; mediastinal windows) from the baseline screening exam of a 67-year-old male current smoker shows a well-defined rounded solid nodule in the right upper lobe. On close inspection, foci of fat can be identified in the nodule's internal matrix. What is the correct Lung-RADS category and appropriate course of management?

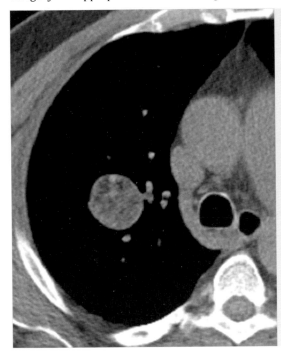

Fig. 10.9 Axial low-dose computed tomography (LDCT) image through the right upper lobe (mediastinal windows) from the baseline screening exam of a 67-year-old man current smoker show a well-defined rounded solid nodule in the right upper lobe. On close inspection, foci of fat can be identified in the nodule's internal matrix.

10.10 Case 10

Axial LDCT image through the upper lung zones from the baseline screening LDCT of a woman with a history of current heavy tobacco abuse shows an 18-mm pure GGN in the anterior segment of the left upper lobe (▶ Fig. 10.10). What is the correct Lung-RADS category and appropriate course of management?

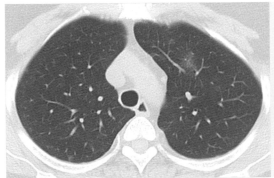

Fig. 10.10 Axial low-dose computed tomography (LDCT) image through the upper lung zones from the baseline screening LDCT of a woman with a history of current heavy tobacco abuse shows an 18-mm pure ground-glass nodule in the anterior segment of the left upper lobe.

10.11 Case Answers

10.11.1 Case 1 Answer

Lung-RADS 4A: Findings for which additional diagnostic testing and/or tissue sampling is recommended, as the probability of potential neoplasia is 5 to 15%. The patient underwent bronchoscopic biopsy that revealed a typical carcinoid tumor. The lesion was subsequently completely removed via endoscopic core and laser without the need for formal thoracotomy.

10.11.2 Case 2 Answer

Lung-RADS 3: Part-solid nodule(s) ≥ 6 mm in total diameter with solid component < 6 mm on baseline imaging. These are probably benign lesions(s); however, short-term follow-up in 6 months with LDCT is suggested for reevaluation. This includes nodules with a low likelihood of becoming a clinically active cancer. The probability of neoplasia is on the order of 1 to 2%.

10.11.3 Case 3 Answer

Lung-RADS 3: Solid nodule(s) ≥ 6 mm but < 8 mm in diameter on baseline imaging. These are probably benign lesions(s); however, short-term follow-up in 6 months with LDCT is suggested for reevaluation. This includes nodules with a low likelihood of becoming a clinically active cancer. The probability of neoplasia is on the order of 1 to 2%.

10.11.4 Case 4 Answer

Lung-RADS 2: Nonsolid nodule(s) or pure GGN less than 20 mm in diameter or baseline imaging. These nodules have a benign appearance or behavior and have a very low likelihood of becoming a clinically active cancer due to their size or lack of growth on follow-up imaging. The probability of malignancy is less than 1%. The appropriate management recommendation is to continue annual screening with LDCT in 12 months. On follow-up 1 year later (not illustrated), the lesion remained stable. No intervention other than continued annual LDCT is needed. The lesion remains categorized as Lung-RADS 2.

10.11.5 Case 5 Answer

The left upper lobe nodule was originally categorized as Lung-RADS 4A—solid nodules ≥ 8 mm but < 15 mm on baseline imaging. A "suspicious" finding for which additional diagnostic testing and/or tissue sampling is recommended. A 3-month follow-up LDCT or positron emission tomography/CT (PET/CT) may be used when there is a ≥ 8-mm solid component. In actuality, the baseline lesion (▶ Fig. 10.5**a**) could have been elevated to Lung-RADS 4X because of the additional findings of polylobulation and spiculation. On the follow-up LDCT (▶ Fig. 10.5**b**), the polylobulation and spiculation have increased and there has been a significant increase in the size of the lesion. The original nodule has grown 80% (18–10 = 8/10 × 100). The lesion is now clearly a Lung-RADS 4X lesion and is highly suspicious. The probability of neoplasia is now greater than 15%. PET/CT and/or tissue sampling now is the most appropriate course of management depending upon the individual's comorbidities. CT-guided biopsy was subsequently performed (not illustrated) and a diagnosis of lung adenocarcinoma established. The lesion was successfully resected via video-assisted thoracoscopic surgery (VATS). The final pathologic diagnosis after resection was minimally invasive adenocarcinoma (MIA). This case illustrates the importance of spiculation and polylobulation as suspicious morphologic findings and the importance of screened individuals closing adhering to the prescribed interval follow-up recommendations laid out in the Lung-RADS management guidelines.

10.11.6 Case 6 Answer

The right upper lobe nodule was originally categorized as Lung-RADS 3—part-solid nodule(s) ≥ 6 mm in total diameter with the solid component < 6 mm on baseline imaging (▶ Fig. 10.6**a**). Lung-RADS 3 lesions are most often benign with a *low likelihood* of becoming a clinically active cancer and a probability of malignancy ranging on the order of 1 to 2%. A 6-month initial follow-up LDCT is the appropriate course of action. However, this case stresses the importance of screened individuals strongly adhering to the prescribed interim follow-up timetable prescribed by the Lung-RADS system, as a *low likelihood* of neoplasia should not be misconstrued as *no likelihood* of neoplasia. This case also stresses the importance of the radiologist to be particularly wary of pericystic lesions and any changes in the morphologic appearance, nodularity, or wall thickness as a potential harbinger of neoplasia in such lesions. On the follow-up 6-month LDCT (▶ Fig. 10.6**b**), the morphologic appearance of this lesion has markedly changed and it is much more suspicious elevating it to a Lung-RADS 4X category. This lesion now warrants additional diagnostic testing with PET/CT and/or tissue sampling. Subsequent CT-guided fine needle aspiration biopsy revealed adenocarcinoma. The lesion was subsequently successfully resected at VATS with a final diagnosis of MIA. Remember, on LDCT, MIA appears as a part-solid nodule. The solid component may vary in size and represents the focus of invasion. Additional imaging features suggestive of invasion on LDCT include the presence of air bronchograms, spiculated or lobulated borders, pleural retraction, and/or a concave notch in the solid component.

10.11.7 Case 7 Answer

Solid noncalcified nodules ≥ 15 mm in diameter on baseline imaging are Lung-RADS 4B lesions. The polylobulated and spiculated borders and the "notches" are additional imaging features suspicious for differential cell growth and neoplasia elevating this lesion to Lung-RADS 4X—a suspicious lesion for which additional diagnostic testing with PET/CT and/or tissue sampling is recommended. The probability of neoplasia is greater than 15%. Subsequent CT-guided biopsy yielded a diagnosis of lung adenocarcinoma.

10.11.8 Case 8 Answer

Solid, noncalcified, rounded nodules ≥ 6 mm but < 8 mm in diameter on baseline screening LDCT are Lung-RADS 3—probably benign lesions with a low likelihood of becoming a clinically active cancer. The probability of neoplasia is 1 to 2%. A 6-month follow-up LDCT is the appropriate course of management. If this nodule remains stable on that follow-up exam and no additional nodules form in the interim, the score can be downgraded to Lung-RADS 2 and annual follow-up LDCT would then be appropriate.

10.11.9 Case 9 Answer

Nodule(s) with specific patterns of calcification: complete, central, popcorn, concentric rings, and/or fat-containing nodules such as that illustrated in Case 9 (p. 96) (▶ Fig. 10.9) are Lung-RADS 1—definitely benign nodules. The appropriate management is annual LDCT and encouraging enrollment in a smoking cessation program.

10.11.10 Case 10 Answer

Pure GGN measuring less than 20 mm in diameter on baseline screens (▶ Fig. 10.10) are nodules with a very low likelihood of becoming a clinically active cancer due to their size or lack of growth on follow-up studies. Such lesions are categorized as Lung-RADS 2 with a probability of neoplasia less than 1%. The appropriate recommendation is continued annual follow-up with LDCT.

Suggested Readings

[1] American College of Radiology. Lung CT Screening Reporting and Data System (Lung-RADS™). Available at: https://www.acr.org/Quality-Safety/Resources/LungRADS

[2] American College of Radiology. Lung-RADS™ Version 1.0 Assessment Categories. 2014. https://www.acr.org/~/media/ACR/Documents/PDF/QualitySafety/Resources/LungRADS/AssessmentCategories.pdf

[3] Rampinelli C, Calloni SF, Minotti M, Bellomi M. Spectrum of early lung cancer presentation in low-dose screening CT: a pictorial review. Insights Imaging. 2016; 7(3):449–459

Index

Note: Page numbers set **bold** or *italic* indicate headings or figures, respectively.